Group Schema Therapy for Complex Trauma

An Evidence-Based Guide to Neuroscience-Informed Group Treatment

Sandoval Sherri Williamson and Ann Ruben McDowell

ISBN: 978-1-7642235-1-5

Isohan Publishing

Table of Contents

Chapter 1: Complex Trauma and Its Neurobiological Impact

The human brain does not distinguish between a tiger in the jungle and a screaming parent in the kitchen. Both activate the same survival circuits, flooding the system with stress hormones and triggering protective responses that can persist long after safety returns. This fundamental reality shapes our understanding of complex trauma—a condition that rewires the nervous system through repeated exposure to overwhelming events, particularly during childhood when the brain remains most malleable.

Complex trauma differs from single-incident posttraumatic stress disorder in both scope and impact. While a car accident or natural disaster might create specific trauma responses tied to that event, complex trauma emerges from chronic, repeated exposure to traumatic situations. The developing brain, faced with ongoing threat, adapts by becoming hypervigilant to danger while struggling to recognize safety when it appears.

Complex Trauma vs. Single-Incident PTSD

Single-incident PTSD typically results from one overwhelming event—a combat experience, sexual assault, or natural disaster. The trauma response centers around that specific incident, with symptoms like intrusive memories, avoidance behaviors, and hyperarousal directly connected to reminders of the original event. Treatment often focuses on processing that singular traumatic experience and reducing its emotional charge.

Complex trauma, however, stems from prolonged, repeated exposure to traumatic events, often occurring in relationships where the victim cannot escape. Childhood abuse, domestic violence, human trafficking, or extended combat exposure create this pattern. The trauma becomes woven into the person's developing sense of self, relationships, and worldview.

Consider Maria, a 34-year-old teacher who entered group therapy after struggling with depression and relationship difficulties. Her childhood included an alcoholic father who alternated between emotional warmth and explosive rage, and a mother who withdrew into depression, leaving Maria to care for her younger siblings. Unlike someone with single-incident PTSD, Maria's trauma symptoms weren't tied to one specific event but to patterns of relationship dynamics, emotional regulation difficulties, and a persistent sense of being responsible for others' well-being.

James presents another example of complex trauma's pervasive effects. Now 28, he experienced sexual abuse by an older cousin from ages 6 to 12, combined with emotional neglect from parents who were physically present but emotionally unavailable. His trauma manifests not as flashbacks to specific incidents but as a generalized fear of intimacy, difficulty trusting his own perceptions, and a tendency to dissociate during emotional conversations.

Developmental Trauma and Attachment Disruption

The timing of trauma exposure significantly affects its impact on development. The human brain undergoes rapid growth during the first three years of life, forming over 700 neural connections per second. During this critical period, children depend entirely on caregivers for safety, regulation, and basic needs. Trauma occurring during these formative years disrupts fundamental developmental processes.

Attachment theory provides the framework for understanding this disruption. Secure attachment develops when caregivers consistently respond to a child's needs with sensitivity and attunement. The child learns that relationships provide safety, that emotions can be managed through connection with others, and that their needs matter. This foundation supports healthy emotional regulation, positive self-concept, and the ability to form trusting relationships throughout life.

Developmental trauma fractures this foundation. Children exposed to abuse, neglect, or chronic family dysfunction develop insecure or disorganized attachment patterns. They may become anxiously attached, constantly seeking reassurance while simultaneously expecting rejection. Others develop avoidant attachment, learning to suppress emotional needs and maintain distance from others. Most concerning is disorganized attachment, where the child experiences the caregiver as both source of comfort and threat, creating internal chaos that persists into adulthood.

Sarah's story illustrates developmental trauma's lasting effects. Born to a mother struggling with bipolar disorder and substance abuse, Sarah experienced periods of intense, overwhelming attention alternating with complete neglect. By age five, she had learned to monitor her mother's moods, becoming hypervigilant to emotional cues while suppressing her own needs. Now 42, Sarah continues this pattern in relationships, becoming anxious when partners seem distant while simultaneously pushing them away when they get too close.

Neurobiological Sequelae

Limbic Dysregulation and Prefrontal Cortex Impairment

Chronic trauma exposure creates measurable changes in brain structure and function. The limbic system, including the amygdala and hippocampus, becomes hyperactive and oversensitive to threat. Meanwhile, the prefrontal cortex—responsible for executive functions like planning, decision-making, and emotional regulation—may become underactive or impaired.

The amygdala serves as the brain's alarm system, constantly scanning for danger. In individuals with complex trauma, this alarm system becomes hypersensitive, firing in response to situations that others might find mildly stressful or completely benign. A raised voice, unexpected touch, or even certain facial expressions can trigger a full threat response.

The hippocampus, responsible for memory formation and contextual learning, also suffers under chronic stress. High levels of cortisol—the primary stress hormone—can actually shrink the hippocampus,

3

impairing the ability to distinguish between past and present experiences. This explains why trauma survivors may react to current situations as if past dangers were happening right now.

The prefrontal cortex, our brain's CEO, struggles to maintain control when the limbic system runs wild. This region, responsible for rational thinking, impulse control, and emotional regulation, requires significant energy and resources to function properly. Under chronic stress, the brain prioritizes survival over higher-order thinking, leaving individuals feeling like passengers in their own lives.

Dr. Bessel van der Kolk's research (1) demonstrates that trauma survivors often show decreased activity in Broca's area—the brain region responsible for speech production—during trauma activation. This neurobiological reality explains why clients often struggle to "just talk about" their experiences. The very act of verbal processing becomes neurologically challenging when trauma responses activate.

The Window of Tolerance and Hyperarousal/Hypoarousal Cycles

Dr. Dan Siegel's concept of the "window of tolerance" (2) provides a useful framework for understanding trauma's impact on nervous system regulation. This window represents the zone where an individual can experience emotions and sensations without becoming overwhelmed or shutting down. Within this zone, people can think clearly, respond flexibly to challenges, and maintain connection with others.

Complex trauma narrows this window significantly. Trauma survivors spend much of their time outside their window of tolerance, oscillating between hyperarousal and hypoarousal states. Hyperarousal manifests as anxiety, panic, rage, hypervigilance, and intrusive thoughts or images. The nervous system runs hot, flooded with stress hormones and primed for fight or flight responses.

Hypoarousal represents the opposite extreme—numbness, depression, dissociation, fatigue, and disconnection from others. The nervous system essentially shuts down to protect against overwhelming stimulation. Neither state allows for optimal functioning or genuine connection with others.

Michael's experience exemplifies these cycles. A 31-year-old veteran who experienced multiple combat deployments, he alternates between periods of explosive anger and emotional numbness. During hyperarousal episodes, minor frustrations—traffic jams, long lines at stores, his children's normal noise levels—trigger intense rage responses. He describes feeling "like a pot about to boil over" during these times. The hypoarousal periods that follow leave him feeling disconnected from his family, going through the motions of daily life without experiencing genuine emotion or pleasure.

Assessment Tools and Differential Diagnosis

Accurate assessment of complex trauma requires understanding its multifaceted presentation. Unlike single-incident PTSD, complex trauma affects multiple domains of functioning: emotional regulation, consciousness, self-concept, relationships, systems of meaning, and behavioral control. Several assessment tools help clinicians identify and measure these effects.

The Adverse Childhood Experiences (ACEs) questionnaire (3) provides a starting point for understanding childhood trauma exposure. This ten-item screening tool identifies experiences of abuse, neglect, and household dysfunction during the first 18 years of life. Research consistently shows that higher ACE scores correlate with increased risk for physical health problems, mental health issues, and social difficulties in adulthood.

However, ACEs alone don't capture the full picture of complex trauma. The Clinician-Administered PTSD Scale for DSM-5 (CAPS-5) (4) offers a structured interview for assessing PTSD symptoms, while the Trauma Symptom Inventory-2 (TSI-2) (5) measures a broader range of trauma-related symptoms including dissociation, sexual concerns, and somatic symptoms.

For complex trauma specifically, the International Trauma Questionnaire (ITQ) (6) assesses symptoms consistent with Complex PTSD as defined in the ICD-11. This instrument measures not only traditional PTSD symptoms but also disturbances in emotional regulation, negative self-concept, and interpersonal difficulties that characterize complex trauma presentations.

The Dissociative Experiences Scale (DES) (7) becomes particularly important when assessing complex trauma survivors, as dissociation frequently accompanies severe or prolonged trauma exposure. Scores above 30 suggest clinically significant dissociative symptoms that require specialized intervention approaches.

Lisa's assessment process illustrates the complexity of trauma evaluation. Initially presenting with depression and relationship difficulties, her ACE score of 8 indicated significant childhood trauma exposure. The CAPS-5 revealed subsyndromal PTSD symptoms—she met criteria for some but not all symptom clusters. However, the ITQ clearly identified complex trauma patterns, including severe emotional dysregulation, persistent negative self-concept, and profound interpersonal difficulties. The DES score of 35 indicated significant dissociative symptoms that explained her "spacing out" during stressful conversations and inability to remember large portions of her childhood.

Differential diagnosis requires careful consideration of comorbid conditions common in complex trauma survivors. Major depressive disorder, anxiety disorders, borderline personality disorder, and substance use disorders frequently co-occur with complex trauma. Rather than viewing these as separate conditions, experienced clinicians recognize them as different expressions of the same underlying trauma-related dysregulation.

The challenge lies in distinguishing complex trauma from other conditions that may present similarly. Borderline personality disorder, for example, shares many features with complex trauma including emotional dysregulation, interpersonal difficulties, and identity disturbance. However, complex trauma typically has clearer connections to specific traumatic experiences and may respond differently to treatment approaches.

Attachment disorders in adults present another diagnostic consideration. While not formally recognized in the DSM-5, many complex trauma survivors struggle with attachment difficulties that significantly impact their relationships and overall functioning. Understanding these patterns helps clinicians develop more effective treatment plans that address the relational aspects of healing.

The assessment process should also consider cultural factors that may influence trauma presentation and help-seeking behaviors. Some cultures emphasize somatic expressions of distress over emotional symptoms, while others may view therapy or mental health treatment with suspicion. Culturally competent assessment recognizes these differences and adapts evaluation approaches accordingly.

Moving Forward: The Foundation for Healing

Understanding complex trauma's neurobiological impact provides the foundation for effective treatment. When clients understand that their symptoms represent normal responses to abnormal circumstances, shame often decreases and hope for healing increases. The brain's neuroplasticity—its ability to form new neural pathways throughout life—offers promise that change remains possible even after years of trauma-related struggling.

This neurobiological perspective also informs treatment approach. Traditional talk therapy alone may prove insufficient for clients whose trauma responses operate below the level of conscious awareness. Effective treatment must address both the cognitive and somatic aspects of trauma, helping clients develop new ways of regulating their nervous systems while processing traumatic experiences.

Group therapy offers unique advantages for complex trauma treatment. The interpersonal nature of complex trauma often requires interpersonal healing. Groups provide opportunities for corrective relational experiences, allowing members to practice new ways of relating while receiving support and feedback from others who understand their struggles.

The assessment process should continue throughout treatment, as trauma symptoms may shift and change as clients develop greater capacity for regulation and integration. What appears as depression or anxiety in early sessions may reveal itself as trauma responses once clients develop language and awareness for their experiences.

Closing Reflections: The Resilience Within

Complex trauma survivors possess remarkable resilience, having developed sophisticated survival strategies that enabled them to endure overwhelming circumstances. These same survival mechanisms that once protected them may now interfere with their ability to thrive in safer environments. Treatment involves honoring these protective strategies while gently helping clients develop new ways of navigating the world.

The journey from survival to thriving requires patience, compassion, and skilled guidance. By understanding the neurobiological foundations of complex trauma, clinicians can offer hope grounded in science while providing interventions that address the whole person—mind, body, and spirit.

Key Learning Points

- Complex trauma results from repeated, prolonged exposure to traumatic events and creates more pervasive effects than single-incident PTSD
- Developmental trauma disrupts attachment formation and creates lasting changes in how individuals relate to themselves and others
- Chronic trauma exposure alters brain structure and function, particularly affecting the limbic system and prefrontal cortex

- The window of tolerance concept explains how trauma survivors oscillate between hyperarousal and hypoarousal states
- Assessment requires multiple tools and consideration of trauma's effects across various domains of functioning
- Understanding trauma's neurobiological impact reduces shame and provides hope for healing through neuroplasticity

Chapter 2: Schema Therapy Model Applied to Complex Trauma

The wounded child within each trauma survivor carries not just memories of what happened, but deeply ingrained beliefs about themselves, others, and the world. These beliefs—what schema therapy calls early maladaptive schemas—form during childhood as adaptive responses to threatening environments but later become rigid patterns that interfere with healthy functioning. Understanding how schemas develop and operate in trauma survivors provides a roadmap for healing that addresses both symptoms and their underlying structure.

Jeffrey Young's schema therapy model (8) offers a framework particularly well-suited for complex trauma treatment. While traditional cognitive-behavioral approaches focus on changing thoughts and behaviors, schema therapy recognizes that trauma creates deeper shifts in core beliefs, emotional patterns, and coping strategies. These schemas operate largely outside conscious awareness, driving reactions and decisions in ways that often perplex both clients and their loved ones.

Early Maladaptive Schemas in Trauma Survivors

Early maladaptive schemas represent stable, pervasive themes about oneself and relationships with others that develop during childhood and persist throughout life. Young identified 18 schemas organized into five domains: disconnection and rejection, impaired autonomy and performance, impaired limits, other-directedness, and overvigilance and inhibition. Trauma survivors typically develop multiple schemas across several domains.

The **abandonment/instability schema** emerges when children experience inconsistent or unreliable caregiving. Adults with this schema constantly fear that significant others will leave them, either emotionally or physically. They may cling desperately to relationships while simultaneously pushing people away through their anxious demands for reassurance.

The **mistrust/abuse schema** develops when children experience betrayal, abuse, or exploitation by those meant to protect them. These individuals expect others to hurt, abuse, manipulate, or take advantage of them. They remain hypervigilant for signs of potential harm, often misinterpreting neutral behaviors as threatening.

The **emotional deprivation schema** forms when children's emotional needs for affection, empathy, or protection remain unmet. Adults with this schema believe that others will never understand or support their emotional needs. They may appear self-sufficient while secretly longing for connection they believe impossible to achieve.

The **defectiveness/shame schema** creates a persistent sense of being flawed, bad, or worthless. Children who experience abuse often internalize blame, concluding that they must be fundamentally defective to deserve such treatment. This schema drives perfectionism, people-pleasing, and avoidance of intimate relationships where perceived flaws might be exposed.

Rachel's story illustrates multiple schema development. At age 38, she struggles with relationships and career advancement despite obvious intelligence and capability. Her childhood included a mother with severe depression who provided little emotional support and a father who was critical and demanding. Rachel developed strong abandonment/instability, emotional deprivation, and defectiveness/shame schemas. In relationships, she becomes anxious when partners seem distant (abandonment schema), doesn't express her emotional needs because she expects disappointment (emotional deprivation schema), and constantly worries that others will discover she's "not good enough" (defectiveness schema).

Schema Modes and Trauma Responses

While schemas represent stable beliefs and patterns, schema modes describe the moment-to-moment emotional and behavioral states that individuals experience. Modes are like different "parts" of the personality that emerge in response to various triggers and situations. Understanding modes helps explain the rapid shifts in emotion and behavior that characterize many trauma survivors.

Young identified four main mode categories: **child modes** (representing different aspects of the authentic self), **dysfunctional parent modes** (internalized critical or demanding voices), **dysfunctional coping modes** (protective strategies that help manage pain but create other problems), and the **healthy adult mode** (the integrated, functional aspect of personality).

Child Modes in Trauma Survivors

The **vulnerable child mode** contains the core emotional pain from childhood trauma. When this mode activates, individuals feel small, helpless, afraid, or overwhelmed. They may experience intense emotions that seem disproportionate to current situations, as past and present collapse together. This mode requires gentle compassion and protection rather than rational discussion or problem-solving.

The **angry child mode** emerges when the vulnerable child's needs were consistently frustrated or ignored. This mode may express rage, throw tantrums (even in adult bodies), or act out destructively. The anger often masks deeper hurt and reflects the child's natural protest against unfair treatment.

The **impulsive/undisciplined child mode** seeks immediate gratification and acts on impulses without considering consequences. Trauma survivors may use this mode to seek pleasure or relief from emotional pain through behaviors like substance use, sexual acting out, or compulsive spending.

Dysfunctional Parent Modes

The **punitive parent mode** represents internalized critical voices that attack, punish, or blame the person for perceived mistakes or inadequacies. This mode often sounds like harsh caregivers from childhood, delivering messages like "you're stupid," "you deserve what happened," or "you should be able to handle this." The punitive parent mode creates shame and interferes with self-compassion.

The **demanding parent mode** sets impossibly high standards and pushes relentlessly toward achievement or perfection. This mode may drive workaholism, perfectionism, or the belief that love must be earned through performance. It often develops in families where acceptance was conditional on meeting high expectations.

Dysfunctional Coping Modes

Trauma survivors develop various coping modes to manage overwhelming emotions and protect themselves from further hurt. While these modes served important protective functions, they often create problems in adult relationships and functioning.

The **detached protector mode** creates emotional distance and avoidance as protection against potential hurt. Individuals in this mode may appear aloof, intellectualizing, or disconnected from emotions. They avoid intimate relationships and emotional vulnerability, trading connection for safety.

The **compliant surrenderer mode** involves giving up one's needs and wants to avoid conflict or abandonment. People in this mode become passive, submissive, and overly focused on pleasing others. They may lose touch with their own preferences and desires, becoming chameleon-like in different relationships.

The **self-aggrandizer mode** protects against vulnerability by creating a false sense of superiority or entitlement. This mode may appear narcissistic or grandiose but actually serves to defend against underlying feelings of defectiveness or inadequacy.

Marcus exemplifies how trauma creates multiple modes. A 29-year-old software engineer, he experienced physical abuse from his father and emotional neglect from his mother. His vulnerable child mode carries terror and sadness from childhood, but he rarely allows others to see this pain. Instead, he typically operates from detached protector mode, keeping relationships superficial and avoiding emotional conversations. When criticized at work, his punitive parent mode activates, delivering harsh self-attacks that would make his father proud. Occasionally, his angry child mode emerges in explosive outbursts that surprise everyone, including himself.

Fight, Flight, Freeze, and Fawn Responses

Trauma responses can be understood through the lens of four primary survival strategies: fight, flight, freeze, and fawn. Each response corresponds to different schema modes and coping strategies, and individuals may use different responses depending on the situation and their perceived options for safety.

The **fight response** activates when individuals perceive threat but believe they have the power to overcome it. This response may manifest as the angry child mode, becoming aggressive, argumentative, or confrontational. While fighting can be adaptive in genuinely dangerous situations, trauma survivors may overuse this response, creating conflict in safe relationships.

The **flight response** emerges when escape seems possible and preferable to confrontation. This might appear as the impulsive child mode, leading to behaviors like substance use, compulsive activities, or literal avoidance of triggering situations. Some individuals develop patterns of leaving relationships or jobs when they become too emotionally intense.

The **freeze response** occurs when neither fight nor flight seems viable. The person becomes immobilized, unable to take action or make decisions. This may manifest as dissociation, depression, or the detached protector mode. Freeze responses often develop in situations where children had no escape from abuse or neglect.

The **fawn response** involves attempting to appease or please the threat source to ensure survival. This response often appears as the compliant surrenderer mode, with individuals becoming overly accommodating, losing their sense of self in relationships, or taking responsibility for others' emotions and behaviors.

Jennifer's trauma responses illustrate this framework clearly. Growing up with an alcoholic, violent father and a mother who couldn't protect her, she learned different strategies for different situations. With her father, she used fawn responses (compliance, people-pleasing) to avoid his wrath. With peers who bullied her at school, she sometimes used fight responses, getting into trouble for aggressive behavior. As an adult, she continues these patterns—fawning with authority figures while fighting with romantic partners when she feels threatened by intimacy.

Coping Strategies: Overcompensation, Avoidance, and Surrender

Schema therapy identifies three primary coping strategies that individuals use to manage schema activation: overcompensation, avoidance, and surrender. Understanding these strategies helps explain seemingly contradictory behaviors in trauma survivors and guides treatment interventions.

Overcompensation involves doing the opposite of what the schema suggests. Someone with a defectiveness schema might become perfectionistic, working relentlessly to prove their worth. A person with an abandonment schema might become the one who leaves first in relationships, attempting to control the inevitable rejection they expect.

Avoidance means staying away from situations that might trigger schema activation. Someone with a mistrust schema might avoid close relationships entirely. A person with a failure schema might avoid taking on new challenges where they could potentially fail.

Surrender involves giving in to the schema, confirming its validity through behavior. Someone with an emotional deprivation schema might choose partners who are emotionally unavailable, unconsciously confirming their belief that their needs won't be met.

Most individuals use all three coping strategies at different times, and the same person might use different strategies for different schemas. This creates complex behavioral patterns that can confuse both the individual and those around them.

The Healthy Adult Mode in Trauma Recovery

The healthy adult mode represents the integrated, functional aspect of personality that can respond to situations with flexibility, wisdom, and appropriate emotional regulation. For trauma survivors, this mode is often underdeveloped or overwhelmed by more dominant trauma-related modes.

The healthy adult mode serves several functions in recovery. It can **nurture the vulnerable child** by providing comfort, validation, and protection when painful emotions arise. It can **set limits with dysfunctional parent modes** by challenging harsh self-criticism or impossible demands. It can **make conscious choices about coping strategies** rather than automatically falling into habitual patterns.

Developing the healthy adult mode becomes a central focus of schema therapy. This involves helping clients recognize their various modes, understand how they developed, and learn to strengthen the healthy adult's capacity to care for wounded parts while making conscious choices about behavior.

Case Conceptualization Framework

Effective schema therapy requires careful case conceptualization that identifies the client's dominant schemas, primary modes, and coping strategies. This framework guides treatment planning and helps therapists understand the client's internal world.

David's case conceptualization illustrates this process. A 35-year-old accountant seeking help for depression and relationship difficulties, David's assessment revealed several key schemas. His abandonment/instability schema developed after his mother's death when he was eight and his father's subsequent emotional withdrawal.

His emotional deprivation schema formed from years of having his grief and needs minimized by well-meaning relatives who told him to "be strong for his father."

David's primary mode pattern involves operating from detached protector mode in most situations, keeping others at arm's length to avoid potential abandonment. When relationships become intimate, his vulnerable child mode emerges with intense fears of being left, triggering clingy behaviors that often push partners away. His punitive parent mode then attacks him for being "needy" and "pathetic," confirming his defectiveness schema.

His primary coping strategy is avoidance—he avoids deep emotional connections, avoids expressing needs, and avoids situations where he might be rejected. Occasionally, he overcompensates by becoming the perfect partner, anticipating and meeting his girlfriend's every need while ignoring his own.

Treatment planning for David focuses on helping him recognize these patterns, develop his healthy adult mode's capacity to nurture his vulnerable child, and gradually practice expressing needs and tolerating the anxiety that comes with emotional risk-taking.

The Therapeutic Relationship as Schema Healing

The therapeutic relationship itself becomes a vehicle for schema healing. Many schemas developed in relationship, and they must be healed in relationship. Therapists provide what Young calls "limited reparenting"—offering the safety, attunement, and care that was missing in childhood while maintaining appropriate professional boundaries.

This process requires therapists to recognize when they're interacting with various client modes and respond accordingly. The vulnerable child mode needs empathy and validation, not interpretation or challenge. The punitive parent mode needs gentle confrontation and limit-setting. The detached protector mode needs patience and consistent, non-intrusive caring.

Integration and Healing

Schema therapy recognizes that healing doesn't mean eliminating schemas or modes entirely. Instead, the goal is integration—helping clients recognize their patterns, understand their origins, and develop choice about how to respond. Schemas may always be present to some degree, but they don't have to control behavior or limit life possibilities.

The process requires patience and compassion, both from therapists and clients themselves. Schemas developed over years or decades don't change quickly. However, with consistent work, clients can develop new experiences that gradually modify old patterns and create possibilities for more satisfying relationships and life experiences.

Moving Toward Wholeness

Schema therapy's strength lies in its recognition that trauma creates coherent, understandable patterns of thinking, feeling, and behaving. These patterns made sense in the contexts where they developed, even if they create problems in current circumstances. By understanding and working with schemas and modes, clients can reclaim parts of themselves that were buried or distorted by trauma while developing new capacities for authentic relationship and self-expression.

The integration of schema therapy principles into group treatment offers additional healing opportunities. Group members can witness each other's modes, provide corrective feedback, and practice new ways of relating in a safe environment. The group becomes a laboratory for experimenting with healthier ways of connecting while processing the schema-driven patterns that have limited their relationships.

Bridging Understanding

Schema therapy provides a bridge between understanding trauma's impact and creating pathways for healing. By recognizing that symptoms represent organized patterns of adaptation rather than random psychological disturbance, both clients and therapists can approach treatment with greater hope and clarity. The next step involves understanding how the nervous system itself responds to trauma and how we can work with these responses to support healing and integration.

Key Learning Points

- Early maladaptive schemas form during childhood as adaptive responses to threatening environments but become rigid patterns that interfere with adult functioning
- Schema modes represent moment-to-moment emotional states that help explain rapid shifts in trauma survivors' emotions and behaviors
- Four primary trauma responses (fight, flight, freeze, fawn) correspond to different schema modes and coping strategies
- Three main coping strategies (overcompensation, avoidance, surrender) explain how individuals manage schema activation
- The healthy adult mode serves as an internal resource for nurturing wounded parts and making conscious behavioral choices
- Case conceptualization identifies dominant schemas, modes, and coping patterns to guide treatment planning
- The therapeutic relationship provides opportunities for limited reparenting and corrective relational experiences

Chapter 3: Polyvagal Theory and Autonomic Nervous System Regulation

The nervous system speaks a language older than words, communicating safety and danger through sensations most people never consciously notice. A slight tightening in the chest, a flutter in the stomach, the urge to look toward an exit—these bodily signals guide our responses to the world around us. For trauma survivors, this ancient communication system often broadcasts danger signals even in safe environments, creating a cascade of reactions that can seem puzzling or overwhelming.

Stephen Porges' polyvagal theory (9) revolutionized our understanding of how the autonomic nervous system responds to safety and threat. Rather than the simple fight-or-flight model many learned in school, polyvagal theory reveals a sophisticated hierarchy of responses that evolved to help mammals survive in social groups. Understanding this hierarchy becomes essential for anyone working with trauma survivors, as their symptoms often represent normal nervous system responses to perceived threat.

Stephen Porges' Polyvagal Theory Fundamentals

The autonomic nervous system operates largely outside conscious awareness, automatically adjusting heart rate, breathing, digestion, and other bodily functions to meet environmental demands. Traditional models divided this system into two branches: the sympathetic (activating) and parasympathetic (calming). Polyvagal theory reveals greater complexity, identifying three distinct circuits that evolved at different points in mammalian development.

The **dorsal vagal complex** represents the oldest evolutionary circuit, shared with reptiles and primitive vertebrates. This system responds to life-threatening situations by shutting down metabolic processes, slowing heart rate, and reducing awareness. In humans, extreme dorsal vagal activation creates dissociation, depression, fainting, or the feeling of being "dead inside."

The **sympathetic nervous system** evolved next, enabling mammals to mobilize energy for fighting or fleeing when faced with danger. This system increases heart rate, breathing, and muscle tension while redirecting blood flow from digestion to major muscle groups. Sympathetic activation creates the familiar fight-or-flight response that helped our ancestors survive predators and other threats.

The **ventral vagal complex** represents the newest evolutionary development, found only in mammals and most sophisticated in primates and humans. This system enables social engagement and calm states conducive to connection, learning, and restoration. When the ventral vagal system is active, people feel safe, curious, and able to engage meaningfully with others.

These three systems operate in a hierarchy, with newer systems inhibiting older ones when conditions allow. The ventral vagal system normally keeps the sympathetic system in check, while sympathetic activation suppresses dorsal vagal responses. However, when the newer systems become overwhelmed or unavailable, older systems take control.

The Neuroception Process

Porges introduced the concept of "neuroception"—the unconscious detection of safety or danger in the environment. Unlike perception, which involves conscious awareness, neuroception operates automatically through sensory pathways that bypass higher brain regions. The nervous system constantly scans for cues of safety, danger, or life threat, adjusting our physiological state accordingly.

Cues of safety include familiar voices with prosodic qualities (melody and rhythm), gentle facial expressions, slow movements, and environmental factors like appropriate lighting and comfortable temperature. When the nervous system detects these cues, the ventral vagal system activates, supporting social engagement and calm alertness.

Cues of danger trigger sympathetic activation and include loud noises, sudden movements, angry voices, unfamiliar environments, or anything reminiscent of past threatening experiences. The sympathetic response prepares the body for action, creating energy and focus needed to address potential threats.

Cues of life threat activate the dorsal vagal system, including situations where neither fight nor flight seems possible. These might include overwhelming pain, inescapable threat, or reminders of past life-threatening experiences. Dorsal activation creates immobilization, dissociation, or collapse.

For trauma survivors, the neuroception process often becomes skewed toward detecting danger and threat. Experiences that others might find mildly stressful or completely neutral may trigger intense nervous system responses. A supervisor's neutral feedback might activate sympathetic fight-or-flight, while a partner's temporary emotional distance could trigger dorsal collapse.

Mapping Autonomic Profiles in Group Members

Understanding each group member's unique autonomic profile helps therapists recognize when interventions might be most effective and when someone needs support returning to their window of tolerance. Autonomic profiling involves identifying individual patterns of activation, common triggers, and preferred regulation strategies.

Sympathetic dominance characterizes individuals who frequently operate in fight-or-flight mode. They may appear anxious, angry, hypervigilant, or constantly "on edge." These group members might interrupt others, argue defensively, or have difficulty sitting still during sessions. Their nervous systems have learned that mobilization equals safety, even in genuinely safe environments.

Dorsal dominance appears in members who frequently shut down or dissociate. They may seem depressed, lethargic, spacey, or emotionally flat. These individuals might have difficulty engaging in group discussions, appear physically collapsed, or report feeling "dead" or "empty" inside. Their nervous systems protect through disconnection rather than mobilization.

Mixed states involve rapid cycling between sympathetic and dorsal activation. These group members might appear volatile, shifting quickly between anger and withdrawal, anxiety and numbness. Their nervous systems struggle to find stability, bouncing between different survival strategies.

Ventral capacity refers to an individual's ability to access and maintain social engagement states. Some trauma survivors retain significant ventral capacity and can often return to calm, connected states with minimal support. Others have very limited access to ventral states and require considerable help developing regulation skills.

Consider Thomas, a 41-year-old combat veteran in group therapy. His autonomic profile shows strong sympathetic dominance—he arrives early to scan the room, sits with his back to the wall, and startles visibly at unexpected sounds. During emotional discussions, his jaw tightens, his breathing becomes shallow, and his voice takes on a hard edge. He reports sleeping 3-4 hours nightly and drinking coffee constantly to maintain alertness. His nervous system interprets most situations as potentially dangerous, keeping him in chronic fight-or-flight activation.

Contrast this with Elena, a 33-year-old survivor of childhood sexual abuse who shows dorsal dominance. She often arrives to group looking exhausted, moves slowly, and speaks in a flat, quiet voice. During intense discussions, she appears to "space out," staring blankly and not responding when addressed directly. She reports feeling "like I'm watching my life through a window" and struggles with chronic depression and fatigue. Her nervous system protects through shutdown rather than activation.

Social Engagement System and Co-Regulation

The social engagement system represents one of polyvagal theory's most important contributions to trauma treatment. This system includes the neural regulation of facial expressions, vocalization, and head movements—the primary ways mammals communicate safety to each other. When the ventral vagal system is active, people naturally engage in behaviors that signal safety: soft eye contact, relaxed facial expressions, prosodic vocalizations, and gentle movements.

Co-regulation describes the process by which one person's regulated nervous system helps regulate another's. Parents naturally co-regulate infants through gentle touch, soothing vocalizations, and calm presence. Adults continue to co-regulate throughout life, though often unconsciously. When someone with strong ventral vagal activation interacts with someone in sympathetic or dorsal states, their regulated presence can help the other person return to safety.

This process becomes particularly important in group therapy settings. Group members can provide co-regulation for each other, creating a collective sense of safety that supports individual healing. However, dysregulated group members can also trigger each other's survival responses, creating contagion effects that require skilled therapeutic intervention.

The therapist's own nervous system state significantly influences the group's overall regulation. A therapist operating from ventral vagal activation—calm, present, and attuned—can help regulate an entire group. Conversely, a therapist in sympathetic activation (anxious, rushed, overwhelmed) or dorsal activation (disconnected, flat, going through motions) may inadvertently dysregulate group members.

Neuroception and Safety Detection in Groups

Group settings present unique challenges for neuroception and safety detection. Multiple people in one room create complex social dynamics that can trigger various nervous system responses. Some group members may feel safer in groups, finding comfort in shared experiences and mutual support. Others may find groups inherently threatening, their nervous systems detecting potential danger in the unpredictability of multiple personalities and emotional states.

Environmental factors significantly influence group neuroception. Room temperature, lighting, seating arrangements, noise levels, and even colors can impact how safe group members feel. Harsh fluorescent lighting might trigger sympathetic responses in some individuals, while dim lighting could feel threatening to others. Circular seating arrangements may feel more connecting to some but more exposing to those who prefer having their backs to walls.

Interpersonal cues constantly influence each member's nervous system state. One person's anxious energy can activate others' sympathetic responses, while someone's calm presence might help others regulate. Facial expressions, tone of voice, body posture, and movement patterns all communicate safety or danger below the level of conscious awareness.

Therapeutic attunement requires therapists to monitor not just the content of what group members share but also their autonomic states and the overall nervous system climate of the group. Recognizing when someone has shifted into sympathetic or dorsal activation allows for timely interventions that support regulation before symptoms become overwhelming.

Sarah's experience illustrates complex group neuroception. Initially, she found the group overwhelming—eight people felt like "too many variables to track," keeping her sympathetic system chronically activated. She positioned herself near the door and frequently checked her watch, seeking escape routes and time orientation. However, as she began recognizing other members' stories in her own experiences, her nervous system gradually detected cues of safety in their shared understanding. The same group that initially felt threatening became a source of regulation and healing.

Autonomic Ladders and Intervention Strategies

Deb Dana's concept of autonomic ladders (10) provides a practical framework for understanding and working with nervous system states. The ladder metaphor helps both therapists and clients visualize movement between different states and identify specific interventions that support upward movement toward ventral safety.

The Dorsal Vagal State sits at the bottom of the ladder, characterized by collapse, disconnection, and immobilization. Interventions at this level focus on gentle re-engagement with the body and environment. Simple breathing exercises, soft music, gentle movement, or warm liquids can help begin the process of moving up the ladder.

The Sympathetic State occupies the middle of the ladder, involving mobilization and activation. Interventions here help discharge excess energy while supporting a sense of agency and control. Physical exercise, bilateral stimulation, rhythmic activities, or expressing anger appropriately can help metabolize sympathetic activation.

The Ventral Vagal State represents the top of the ladder, characterized by safety, connection, and social engagement. Interventions support maintaining this state through practices like mindful breathing, gentle yoga, creative expression, meaningful conversation, or activities that promote flow states.

Understanding that movement up the ladder typically occurs gradually helps set realistic expectations for both therapists and clients. Someone in deep dorsal collapse cannot immediately access ventral connection—they must first move through sympathetic activation. This explains why some trauma survivors may appear to get "worse" before getting better, as they begin feeling emotions and sensations that were previously shut down.

Glimmers represent brief moments of ventral activation that can be cultivated and expanded over time. These might include the warmth felt when a pet curls up nearby, the satisfaction of completing a task, or the connection experienced during a meaningful conversation. Learning to notice and nurture glimmers helps build ventral capacity gradually.

Triggers represent stimuli that rapidly shift someone down the autonomic ladder toward sympathetic or dorsal states. Identifying personal triggers helps individuals develop strategies for managing these shifts and returning to regulation more quickly.

Marcus learned to recognize his movement down the autonomic ladder through body awareness. When stressed, he first noticed his jaw clenching and shoulders rising—early signs of sympathetic activation. If he didn't address these cues, his breathing would become shallow, his thoughts would race, and he'd begin snapping at colleagues. Eventually, if the stress continued, he'd crash into dorsal collapse, feeling exhausted and disconnected from everyone around him.

By learning to recognize these patterns, Marcus developed intervention strategies for each state. Early sympathetic activation responded well to brief walks, deep breathing, or calling a supportive friend. More intense sympathetic states required physical exercise or progressive muscle relaxation. When he caught himself sliding toward dorsal collapse, gentle music, warm tea, and reading helped him gradually re-engage.

Polyvagal-Informed Group Interventions

Group therapy offers unique opportunities for polyvagal-informed interventions that leverage the power of co-regulation and social engagement. These interventions work with the nervous system rather than against it, supporting natural healing processes rather than forcing change through willpower alone.

Regulation check-ins at the beginning of each group session help members and therapists assess current autonomic states. Simple questions like "How is your nervous system feeling today?" or "What do you notice in your body right now?" promote awareness while providing information about who might need additional support.

Breathing exercises performed together create opportunities for co-regulation while supporting ventral activation. Group breathing doesn't require everyone to breathe identically but rather creates a shared rhythm that can help regulate individual nervous systems.

Movement and rhythm activities engage the social engagement system through shared physical experiences. Simple movements like gentle stretching, walking meditation, or even coordinated hand movements can help group members feel more connected to their bodies and each other.

Vocal exercises work directly with the social engagement system through the neural pathways that connect the heart, larynx, and middle ear. Humming, chanting, or singing together can activate ventral pathways while creating group cohesion.

Mindful observation helps group members practice neuroception awareness by noticing environmental cues of safety and danger. This might involve identifying what makes the group room feel safe or discussing how different members' presence affects their nervous systems.

Working with Autonomic Mismatches

Group members often experience autonomic states that don't match their conscious intentions or the group's current focus. Someone might want to engage in emotional processing while their nervous system remains in dorsal shutdown. Another member might intellectually understand that the group is safe while their sympathetic system continues scanning for threats.

These mismatches require patience and understanding rather than pressure to change. Acknowledging autonomic states validates group members' experiences while reducing shame about their responses. "It makes sense that your nervous system is protecting you right now" normalizes trauma responses while opening possibilities for gentle movement toward regulation.

Sometimes group members need permission to honor their autonomic states rather than fighting against them. Someone in dorsal collapse might need to listen quietly rather than actively participate. A member in sympathetic activation might need to stand or move during discussions rather than forcing stillness.

Integration and Daily Life Application

The ultimate goal of polyvagal-informed work involves helping group members recognize their autonomic patterns and develop portable regulation strategies for daily life. This requires moving beyond symptom management toward nervous system literacy— understanding how their bodies respond to various situations and what interventions support their unique needs.

Daily practice becomes essential for building ventral capacity and resilience. Just as physical exercise strengthens muscles over time, consistent attention to nervous system regulation gradually expands the window of tolerance and increases access to social engagement states.

Group members often benefit from creating personal regulation toolkits—collections of strategies that work specifically for their nervous systems and life circumstances. These might include breathing techniques, movement practices, environmental modifications, social connection strategies, or sensory tools that support regulation.

Building Resilience Through Understanding

Polyvagal theory offers hope grounded in biology. Understanding that trauma responses represent adaptive nervous system strategies rather than character defects or personal failures reduces shame while increasing possibilities for healing. The nervous system's capacity for change throughout life means that even deeply ingrained patterns can shift with appropriate support and practice.

Group therapy provides an ideal setting for nervous system healing because trauma often occurs in relational contexts and requires relational repair. Group members can practice new ways of being with others while receiving feedback about their impact and presence. The group becomes a safe laboratory for experimenting with vulnerability, connection, and authentic self-expression.

Summary Thoughts

The wisdom of the nervous system extends far beyond simple fight-or-flight responses. Polyvagal theory reveals the sophisticated ways our bodies assess safety and respond to threat, offering roadmaps for healing that honor both individual differences and universal human needs for connection and safety. Understanding these patterns provides the foundation for effective trauma treatment that works with the body's natural healing capacity rather than against it.

Key Learning Points

- Polyvagal theory identifies three evolutionary circuits: dorsal vagal (shutdown), sympathetic (mobilization), and ventral vagal (social engagement)
- Neuroception involves unconscious detection of safety, danger, or life threat that automatically adjusts our physiological state
- Individual autonomic profiles help therapists recognize regulation patterns and tailor interventions accordingly
- Co-regulation through the social engagement system allows regulated individuals to help others return to safety
- Autonomic ladders provide frameworks for understanding movement between nervous system states and planning interventions
- Group settings offer unique opportunities for polyvagal-informed interventions that leverage collective regulation
- Building nervous system literacy helps individuals develop portable regulation strategies for daily life

Chapter 4: The Therapeutic Rationale for Group Treatment

Individual therapy offers privacy and focused attention, but healing from complex trauma often requires something more—the messy, unpredictable, profoundly human experience of genuine connection with others who understand. Groups mirror the interpersonal contexts where trauma typically occurs, providing opportunities for corrective experiences that individual therapy cannot replicate. The very dynamics that initially feel threatening in group settings often become the pathways through which the deepest healing occurs.

The decision to recommend group therapy for complex trauma survivors requires careful consideration of both benefits and risks. Groups can accelerate healing through shared understanding and mutual support, but they can also retraumatize individuals if not carefully structured and skillfully facilitated. Understanding the therapeutic rationale for group treatment helps clinicians make informed decisions about when and how to utilize this powerful modality.

Cost-Effectiveness and Accessibility Benefits

Mental healthcare costs continue rising while insurance coverage becomes increasingly restrictive. Group therapy offers a practical solution that makes intensive trauma treatment accessible to more individuals while maintaining therapeutic effectiveness. The economics matter not just for healthcare systems but for clients who often struggle with employment instability and financial stress as consequences of their trauma histories.

Research consistently demonstrates that group therapy produces outcomes comparable to individual therapy for many conditions, including PTSD and complex trauma (11). When considering cost per therapeutic contact hour, groups provide significantly more value—a 90-minute group session with eight members offers 720 minutes of therapeutic exposure (8 members × 90 minutes) compared to 50 minutes in individual therapy, at roughly comparable cost to the individual session.

However, the accessibility benefits extend beyond simple economics. Many trauma survivors feel more comfortable beginning treatment in groups where they can observe others sharing similar experiences before exposing their own vulnerabilities. The presence of other group members can reduce the intensity of the therapeutic relationship, making it feel less threatening for individuals who struggle with authority figures or intimate relationships.

Geographic accessibility also improves through group treatment. Rural areas with limited mental health resources can serve more trauma survivors through group programs. Online group platforms expand access further, connecting individuals who might otherwise have no access to specialized trauma treatment.

Michelle's story illustrates these accessibility benefits. Living in a small town with one overbooked trauma therapist, she waited eight months for individual therapy. When the therapist offered a trauma group, Michelle initially felt disappointed—she wanted individual attention for her "special" problems. However, the group began three weeks later, providing immediate access to treatment. Moreover, her job in retail management made weekly individual appointments difficult, but the group met in the evenings when she could consistently attend.

Corrective Interpersonal Experiences

Complex trauma typically occurs within relationships—childhood abuse by caregivers, domestic violence by partners, betrayal by trusted others. These experiences create expectations about relationships that persist long after the original trauma ends. Victims learn that relationships involve danger, that their needs don't matter, that others will inevitably hurt or abandon them.

Group therapy provides opportunities to test these beliefs in a controlled, supportive environment. Group members can experience being heard without being judged, receiving support without owing something in return, and expressing anger without being attacked or abandoned. These corrective experiences gradually challenge trauma-based assumptions about relationships.

The interpersonal learning that occurs in groups cannot be replicated in individual therapy. While therapists can discuss relationship patterns, group members actually experience different ways of relating. They practice setting boundaries, expressing needs, giving and receiving feedback, and negotiating conflicts—all while receiving support and guidance from both facilitators and peers.

Power dynamics play out differently in groups than in individual therapy. The therapist's authority becomes diluted among multiple participants, reducing the intensity that some trauma survivors find threatening. Group members often accept feedback from peers more readily than from authority figures, finding validation in shared experiences rather than professional interpretations.

Trust development occurs gradually through multiple small interactions rather than the intense focus of individual therapy. Members can observe how others handle vulnerability and decide how much they want to share. This process respects the protective mechanisms that trauma survivors have developed while creating opportunities for gradual risk-taking.

Intimacy tolerance can be practiced at different levels simultaneously. While one member shares deeply emotional content, another might participate simply by listening attentively. The group accommodates different comfort levels with closeness while providing models of healthy intimacy.

Kevin's experience demonstrates corrective relationship patterns. Growing up with an alcoholic mother who alternated between emotional intimacy and rage, he learned that closeness inevitably led to hurt. In individual therapy, he maintained polite distance from his therapist, discussing problems intellectually while avoiding emotional connection. The group initially felt overwhelming—too many unpredictable people with too many emotions.

However, the group's predictable structure and clear boundaries gradually felt safer than the chaotic intimacy of his childhood. When Sarah cried about her divorce, other members offered support without trying to fix or minimize her pain. When Marcus expressed anger about his boss, no one attacked him or shut him down. Slowly, Kevin began recognizing that emotional expression didn't automatically lead to chaos or attack.

Witnessing and Universality Factors

Irving Yalom identified universality as one of the primary therapeutic factors in group therapy (12)—the recognition that others share similar struggles, reducing shame and isolation. For trauma survivors, this universality becomes particularly powerful because trauma often creates profound feelings of being different, damaged, or alone.

Shame reduction occurs when group members recognize that their responses to trauma are normal and understandable. Hearing others describe similar symptoms, reactions, or struggles helps normalize experiences that felt abnormal or crazy when endured in isolation. The shame that often compounds trauma begins dissolving in the light of shared understanding.

Witnessing provides both therapeutic benefits for those who share and those who listen. Being witnessed in pain by others who understand creates profound validation that cannot be replicated through individual therapy. Simultaneously, witnessing others' stories helps group members gain perspective on their own experiences and recognize their own strength and resilience.

Hope installation develops as group members observe others at different stages of recovery. Newer members can see that healing is possible by watching more experienced members demonstrate healthier coping strategies and improved relationships. Long-term members reinforce their own progress by helping newcomers and recognizing how far they've traveled.

The power of witnessing extends beyond verbal sharing. Group members witness each other's nonverbal expressions, emotional reactions, and behavioral patterns. This comprehensive witnessing helps individuals recognize aspects of themselves they might not consciously notice while feeling seen and understood at deeper levels.

Janet's experience illustrates witnessing power. For years, she believed her reactions to childhood sexual abuse were excessive and abnormal. She criticized herself for struggling with intimacy, having difficulty trusting others, and experiencing anxiety in everyday situations. When she joined the trauma group, she discovered that every member struggled with similar issues.

Listening to Robert describe his hypervigilance in public places, she recognized her own constant scanning for exits and potential threats. Hearing Lisa talk about feeling "dirty" and unworthy of love resonated with her own self-perceptions. Most importantly, seeing how compassionately group members responded to each other's pain helped her begin extending that same compassion to herself.

Group as Microcosm of Family-of-Origin Dynamics

Groups naturally recreate family-of-origin dynamics, providing opportunities to recognize and change dysfunctional patterns in real-time. Members unconsciously assume familiar roles—the caretaker, the scapegoat, the peacemaker, the rebel—while others trigger responses based on past relationships. These dynamics, initially challenging, become valuable material for therapeutic work.

Transference patterns emerge more clearly in groups than individual therapy. Members may react to each other based on past relationships rather than current reality. Someone might feel inexplicably angry at a group member who reminds them of an abusive sibling, or become anxiously attached to someone who resembles a lost parent. These reactions provide direct access to unconscious patterns that might take months to identify in individual therapy.

Role flexibility becomes possible as group members experiment with different ways of being. Someone who always played the family caretaker can practice expressing their own needs. A former family scapegoat can experience being valued and supported. These new roles feel risky initially but become integrated through repeated positive experiences.

Authority relationships play out with group facilitators, allowing members to work through patterns with parental figures. Some members may initially idealize therapists, seeking the perfect parent they never had. Others might be suspicious or oppositional, expecting betrayal or control. These reactions provide valuable information about attachment patterns while offering opportunities for corrective experiences with healthy authority figures.

Sibling dynamics emerge between group members, recreating competition, jealousy, alliance-building, and support patterns from childhood. Unlike family relationships, however, group dynamics can be discussed openly and changed consciously. Members can recognize when they're competing for the therapist's attention and explore what drives this pattern.

David's family dynamics illustrate this process. The oldest of four children with depressed, overwhelmed parents, he learned early to suppress his own needs while managing his siblings' behaviors and emotions. In the group, he automatically assumed the caretaker role, offering advice and support while rarely expressing his own struggles.

Other members began pointing out this pattern, noting how David deflected attention when they tried to support him. The group became a laboratory for practicing receiving care rather than just providing it. When David finally broke down describing his loneliness and exhaustion, the group's supportive response contradicted his childhood experience of being needed only for what he could provide others.

Research Evidence and Outcome Studies

Empirical support for group therapy in trauma treatment continues growing, with studies demonstrating effectiveness across various populations and trauma types. Understanding this research helps clinicians make evidence-based decisions about group treatment while providing clients with realistic expectations about potential outcomes.

Meta-analytic studies consistently show group therapy effectiveness for PTSD treatment comparable to individual approaches. A 2016 meta-analysis found effect sizes ranging from 0.85 to 1.20 for group treatments, indicating large therapeutic effects (13). These studies included diverse populations including veterans, sexual assault survivors, childhood abuse survivors, and mixed trauma groups.

Complex trauma research specifically examining group approaches shows promising results. Studies of group schema therapy for personality disorders demonstrate significant improvements in emotional regulation, interpersonal functioning, and overall symptom reduction (14). While fewer studies examine group schema therapy specifically for complex trauma, available research suggests comparable benefits to individual treatment with additional interpersonal learning opportunities.

Dropout rates in trauma groups vary widely depending on population, treatment approach, and group structure. Well-structured groups with careful screening typically show dropout rates between 15-25%, comparable to individual trauma therapy. Higher dropout rates often reflect inadequate preparation, poor group composition, or insufficient attention to safety and stabilization.

Long-term outcomes appear particularly promising for group approaches. Follow-up studies suggest that gains from group therapy may be better maintained than individual therapy gains, possibly due to continued social support networks that develop during treatment. Group members often maintain informal connections after formal treatment ends, providing ongoing support for continued healing.

Cost-effectiveness studies consistently favor group approaches when considering healthcare utilization, quality of life improvements, and sustained treatment gains. While initial setup costs may be higher due to screening and preparation requirements, the long-term economic benefits support group treatment as a preferred approach for many trauma survivors.

Sandra's outcome illustrates research findings. She completed a 24-week group therapy program for complex trauma after years of struggling with depression, anxiety, and relationship difficulties. Pre-treatment measures showed severe symptoms across multiple domains. Post-treatment assessments revealed significant improvements in emotional regulation, interpersonal relationships, and overall functioning.

More importantly, 18-month follow-up showed maintained gains with continued improvement in several areas. Sandra credited ongoing connections with two group members for providing support during difficult periods. She also reported increased confidence in forming new relationships, partly due to the successful relationships developed during group treatment.

Specialized Group Approaches for Complex Trauma

Different group therapy models offer varying approaches to complex trauma treatment. Understanding these options helps clinicians match treatment approaches to client needs and preferences while considering available resources and expertise.

Process groups focus on here-and-now interactions between members, using group dynamics as the primary therapeutic tool. These groups work well for individuals with good verbal skills and some emotional regulation capacity who can benefit from interpersonal learning. Process groups require significant facilitator skill in managing group dynamics and individual needs simultaneously.

Psychoeducational groups emphasize learning about trauma, coping skills, and recovery strategies. These groups feel safer for many trauma survivors initially because they focus on information rather than emotional sharing. However, they may not provide sufficient opportunities for emotional processing and interpersonal learning that characterize effective trauma treatment.

Skills-based groups teach specific techniques for managing trauma symptoms, such as emotion regulation, mindfulness, or communication skills. These groups work well combined with individual therapy or as preparation for more intensive group work. They provide concrete tools while building confidence and group comfort.

Trauma-focused process groups combine elements of education, skills training, and process work. Members learn about trauma while also processing their experiences and working with group dynamics. This approach provides comprehensive treatment while maintaining focus on trauma-specific issues.

Schema therapy groups specifically address the core beliefs and patterns that develop from childhood trauma. These groups combine psychoeducation about schemas and modes with experiential exercises and interpersonal process work. The structured approach helps contain difficult emotions while providing frameworks for understanding and changing dysfunctional patterns.

Timing and Readiness Considerations

Not all trauma survivors are ready for group therapy at all times. Determining readiness requires careful assessment of current functioning, symptom severity, and individual circumstances. Premature group placement can retraumatize vulnerable individuals, while delayed referral might deprive clients of beneficial treatment.

Stabilization requirements vary among different group approaches. Highly structured psychoeducational groups may accommodate individuals with active symptoms and limited regulation skills. Intensive process groups typically require greater emotional stability and some capacity for self-soothing when activated.

Motivation and commitment become particularly important in group settings where individual absence affects other members. Clients need genuine motivation for change rather than external pressure from others. They also need ability to commit to consistent attendance and group confidentiality.

Social anxiety considerations require balance between honoring protective mechanisms and encouraging therapeutic risk-taking. Some social anxiety actually decreases in groups as individuals recognize shared struggles. However, severe social phobia might require individual preparation before group participation.

Current life stability affects group readiness significantly. Individuals experiencing active crises, major life transitions, or unstable living situations may have difficulty focusing on group process. However, groups can also provide stability and support during challenging periods.

Contraindications and Risk Factors

While group therapy offers significant benefits for many trauma survivors, certain factors increase risks or contraindicate group treatment. Recognizing these factors protects both individual clients and group integrity.

Active psychosis or severe dissociation can interfere with group participation and trigger other members. Individuals need sufficient reality testing and present-moment awareness to participate safely in group discussions.

Severe personality disorders with limited treatment motivation or insight may disrupt group functioning. However, motivated individuals with personality disorders often benefit significantly from group treatment with appropriate structure and limits.

Active substance abuse interferes with emotional processing and group safety. Most groups require sobriety or stable recovery, though some specialized groups work specifically with dual diagnosis clients.

Suicidal ideation or self-harm behaviors require careful assessment. Groups can provide additional support and monitoring, but active suicidality might overwhelm group resources and trigger other members.

Severe aggression or impulse control problems pose safety risks that most groups cannot manage appropriately. Individual treatment focusing on safety and control typically needs to precede group participation.

Integration With Other Treatments

Group therapy works best as part of comprehensive treatment rather than standalone intervention. Understanding how groups integrate with other treatment modalities maximizes therapeutic benefits while addressing individual needs that groups cannot meet.

Individual therapy provides opportunities for deeper exploration of personal issues, crisis intervention, and preparation for group participation. Many clients benefit from concurrent individual and group treatment, using each modality to support the other.

Medication management often becomes necessary for trauma survivors with severe symptoms. Groups can provide support for medication adherence and feedback about effectiveness while individual providers monitor medical needs.

Family therapy may be needed to address current relationship issues that affect recovery. Groups provide practice grounds for new relationship skills while family therapy addresses specific system changes.

Other group experiences like support groups, twelve-step programs, or activity groups can complement trauma therapy groups. However, too many concurrent groups might overwhelm individuals or create conflicting messages about recovery.

Moving Forward Together

Group therapy for complex trauma offers unique healing opportunities that individual treatment cannot replicate. The interpersonal learning, corrective experiences, and mutual support available in groups address the relational aspects of trauma that often maintain symptoms and interfere with recovery. While not appropriate for everyone at all times, groups provide cost-effective, accessible treatment that can accelerate healing for many trauma survivors.

The research supporting group approaches continues growing, providing evidence-based rationale for recommending this treatment modality. However, the real evidence comes from witnessing the transformation that occurs when isolated, shame-filled individuals discover they are not alone, not broken, and not beyond healing. Groups create communities of healing where individual recovery becomes shared triumph.

Essential Insights

- Group therapy provides cost-effective, accessible trauma treatment with outcomes comparable to individual therapy
- Corrective interpersonal experiences in groups challenge trauma-based assumptions about relationships
- Witnessing and universality factors reduce shame and isolation while installing hope for recovery
- Groups recreate family-of-origin dynamics, providing opportunities to recognize and change dysfunctional patterns
- Research evidence consistently supports group approaches for various trauma populations and types
- Different group models offer varying approaches that can be matched to individual needs and readiness levels
- Careful screening and timing considerations ensure appropriate group placement and minimize risks

Chapter 5: Creating Safety and Trust in Trauma Groups

Safety is not merely the absence of danger—it is the embodied sense that one can be authentic without fear of attack, abandonment, or betrayal. For trauma survivors, this feeling may be entirely foreign, a theoretical concept they've heard about but never experienced. Creating genuine safety in trauma groups requires more than establishing rules and boundaries; it demands understanding how traumatized nervous systems detect and respond to threat, then systematically building conditions that support regulation and trust.

The paradox of trauma group formation lies in this reality: the very people who most need safe relationships often find it most difficult to trust others. Their survival has depended on hypervigilance, control, and emotional distance. Asking them to sit in a circle with strangers and share their most vulnerable experiences challenges every protective mechanism they've developed. Success requires patience, skill, and deep appreciation for the courage required to heal in community.

Physical and Psychological Safety Protocols

Creating safety begins with the most basic elements—physical environment, clear structures, and predictable routines that help dysregulated nervous systems recognize they are not in immediate danger. Trauma survivors' neuroception processes constantly scan for threats, often detecting danger in neutral situations. Environmental design can either support or undermine this automatic safety assessment.

Physical environment considerations extend beyond basic comfort to include factors that specifically impact traumatized individuals. Room layout affects safety perceptions significantly—members need clear sight lines to exits, comfortable personal space, and seating arrangements that don't make anyone feel trapped or exposed. Harsh lighting, sudden noises, or uncomfortable temperatures can trigger sympathetic nervous system activation that interferes with therapeutic engagement.

The group room should remain consistent whenever possible, as frequent location changes can activate anxiety in individuals who cope through environmental control and predictability. Comfortable, stable seating helps members feel grounded, while adequate climate control prevents additional stress that might push already-vulnerable nervous systems beyond their windows of tolerance.

Temporal safety involves maintaining consistent meeting times, predictable session structure, and reliable facilitator presence. Trauma survivors often struggle with time perception and may become anxious about late starts, unexpected schedule changes, or ambiguous ending times. Clear communication about any necessary changes, provided as far in advance as possible, respects members' need for predictability and control.

Interpersonal safety protocols establish clear expectations about how group members will treat each other and what behaviors are acceptable within the group. These guidelines go beyond basic confidentiality to address trauma-specific concerns like respecting personal space, avoiding unsolicited advice or problem-solving, and understanding that healing happens at different paces for different people.

The principle of **voluntary participation** becomes essential in trauma groups. Members must feel they can choose their level of engagement in any given session without pressure or judgment. This might mean listening quietly when others share, participating verbally when ready, or taking breaks when overwhelmed. Forced participation can retraumatize individuals whose original trauma involved powerlessness and lack of choice.

Emotional safety boundaries include agreements about not attacking or judging other members, respecting different viewpoints and experiences, and understanding that strong emotional reactions are normal and acceptable. These boundaries help create the psychological holding environment necessary for trauma processing while preventing retraumatization through group interactions.

Jennifer's initial group experience illustrates safety protocol importance. A survivor of childhood physical and sexual abuse, she arrived at her first session twenty minutes early to scope out the room and choose a seat with her back to the wall and clear view of the door. The facilitator's warm but non-intrusive greeting helped her nervous system recognize the therapist as safe, while the predictable check-in structure gave her time to assess other members before deciding how much to participate.

During the third session, another member raised his voice while expressing anger about his ex-wife. Jennifer immediately dissociated, spacing out and becoming unable to track the conversation. The facilitator noticed her absence and gently brought her back to the present, acknowledging that loud voices can be triggering and checking in about what she needed to feel safe. This intervention demonstrated that the group could contain strong emotions without becoming chaotic or dangerous.

Group Composition and Screening Criteria

Thoughtful group composition significantly impacts safety, cohesion, and therapeutic outcomes. While diversity in experiences and backgrounds can enrich group learning, certain combinations of trauma histories, personality styles, or current functioning levels may create dynamics that interfere with healing or compromise safety for vulnerable members.

Trauma type considerations require balancing homogeneous and heterogeneous composition. Groups composed entirely of survivors of the same trauma type (all childhood sexual abuse survivors, all combat veterans) may provide deeper understanding and less need for explanation, but they can also limit perspective and become stuck in shared assumptions or patterns.

Mixed trauma groups offer broader perspectives and reduce the sense that one type of trauma is "worse" than others, but they require more skilled facilitation to ensure all members feel understood and validated. The key lies in ensuring that all members share the common thread of complex trauma, regardless of specific experiences that created it.

Symptom severity matching helps ensure that group members can engage at similar levels without overwhelming each other. Mixing individuals with very different functioning levels can create dynamics where higher-functioning members become frustrated with those struggling more, while lower-functioning members feel inadequate or ashamed of their limitations.

However, some diversity in healing stages can provide hope and modeling for newer members while reinforcing progress for those further along in recovery. The ideal balance includes members at different points in their healing journey but within a range that allows mutual support and understanding.

Personality considerations become particularly important in trauma groups where interpersonal difficulties often represent core treatment targets. Including too many individuals with severe personality disorders, active addiction, or limited insight can overwhelm group resources and interfere with treatment for all members.

Conversely, groups composed entirely of highly functional, insightful individuals may lack the interpersonal challenge necessary for growth and change. Some personality diversity encourages group members to practice new ways of relating while providing opportunities to work through triggered responses in real time.

Motivation and readiness assessment ensures that potential members genuinely want to participate in group treatment rather than attending due to external pressure or crisis intervention needs. Group therapy requires sustained commitment and willingness to engage with others, qualities that may be absent in individuals seeking quick fixes or attending involuntarily.

The screening process should assess potential members' capacity for group participation, including ability to sit through 90-minute sessions, tolerate others' emotional expression, maintain basic behavioral control, and respect confidentiality requirements. These capacities may be temporarily impaired during crisis periods but should be generally available to potential group members.

Marcus's screening process demonstrates thoughtful composition decisions. Initially referred for group therapy immediately following his wife's sudden death, Marcus was clearly in acute grief and crisis. The therapist recognized that while Marcus might eventually benefit from group treatment, his current emotional intensity and crisis state would likely overwhelm him and potentially other group members.

Instead, the therapist recommended individual therapy for crisis stabilization and grief processing, with group therapy as a future option once the acute crisis resolved. Six months later, Marcus joined a mixed trauma group where his experience of sudden loss complemented other members' histories of childhood trauma, providing diverse perspectives while maintaining the common thread of complex trauma responses.

Establishing Group Norms and Boundaries

Clear norms and boundaries provide the structure necessary for psychological safety while establishing expectations that support therapeutic progress. These agreements go beyond basic rules to create a culture of respect, authenticity, and mutual support that facilitates healing. Effective norms are developed collaboratively with group input while maintaining therapeutic structure and safety.

Confidentiality agreements form the foundation of group safety, but trauma survivors often need more detailed explanation about what confidentiality means and why it matters. Standard confidentiality requirements—not sharing what others say outside the group—may need expansion to include not sharing information with other group members outside of sessions, avoiding social media connections, and understanding the limits of confidentiality in situations involving safety concerns.

The concept of **emotional confidentiality** extends beyond information sharing to include not judging, analyzing, or discussing other members' experiences outside of group sessions. This deeper level of respect helps create the safe holding environment necessary for vulnerability and emotional processing.

Communication guidelines help establish how group members will interact with each other, particularly during emotionally charged moments. These might include speaking directly to each other rather than through the facilitator, using "I" statements to express personal reactions, avoiding advice-giving unless requested, and respecting others' right to their own experiences and feelings.

The guideline to **speak from personal experience** rather than making generalizations or assumptions helps group members stay grounded in their own reality while avoiding triggering others through projections or interpretations. This boundary becomes particularly important in trauma groups where members may be sensitive to feeling analyzed or judged.

Attendance expectations balance the need for commitment and predictability with recognition that trauma survivors may struggle with consistency due to symptom flares, dissociation, or other trauma-related difficulties. Reasonable expectations might include notifying the group about planned absences, attending at least 75% of sessions, and discussing attendance problems in group rather than simply disappearing.

Physical boundaries address trauma survivors' often-complicated relationships with touch, personal space, and physical comfort. Clear agreements about no uninvited touch, respecting personal space preferences, and checking before offering comfort through physical contact help prevent inadvertent triggering while allowing for appropriate support when desired.

Time boundaries include starting and ending sessions punctually, respecting speaking time limits to ensure everyone has opportunities to participate, and understanding that crisis processing outside of group time should involve individual therapists or crisis resources rather than other group members.

Sarah's experience with boundary development illustrates collaborative norm-setting. During the second group session, another member offered to hug Sarah after she shared about feeling disconnected from her children. Sarah froze, unable to say no but feeling panicked about unwanted touch. The facilitator intervened gently, suggesting the group discuss how they wanted to handle physical comfort and support.

The resulting conversation led to agreements about always asking permission before offering physical comfort, respecting "no" without taking it personally, and understanding that someone's comfort level might change from session to session. Sarah felt relieved that her trauma response became an opportunity for the group to develop better boundaries rather than evidence of her being "difficult" or "damaged."

Managing Triggers and Re-traumatization Risks

Despite careful preparation and boundary-setting, triggers inevitably occur in trauma groups. The goal is not to prevent all triggering experiences—which would be impossible and therapeutically counterproductive—but to create systems for recognizing, containing, and processing triggers safely when they arise. This requires both preventive strategies and responsive interventions.

Trigger identification and sharing helps group members recognize their own activation patterns while alerting others to potentially sensitive topics or behaviors. This process should be voluntary and ongoing, as trigger awareness often develops gradually through group experience. Members might share that they become activated by angry voices, detailed abuse descriptions, or discussions of certain topics without needing to explain their entire trauma history.

Creating **signal systems** allows group members to communicate their internal state without disrupting the group process. Simple hand signals might indicate "I'm triggered but okay," "I need a break," or "I'm dissociating and need help grounding." These systems respect the reality that triggered individuals may lose capacity for verbal communication while still enabling them to advocate for their needs.

Grounding techniques readily available during group sessions help members manage activation when it occurs. These might include bilateral stimulation tools, stress balls, weighted blankets, essential oils, or other sensory resources that support nervous system regulation. Having these tools visible and accessible normalizes their use while providing immediate support when needed.

The **pause and breathe** intervention allows facilitators to slow down group process when they notice activation spreading among members or when individual members appear overwhelmed. Rather than pushing through difficult material, this intervention creates space for regulation and conscious choice about how to proceed.

Titrated exposure involves helping group members approach difficult topics gradually rather than diving into overwhelming material. This might mean discussing feelings about trauma before sharing specific details, or processing current triggers before exploring their historical origins. Titration respects the nervous system's capacity for integration while still allowing for therapeutic progress.

Processing protocols for when triggers occur include immediate safety assessment, offering choices about continuing participation, providing grounding support, and following up in subsequent sessions to ensure integration and learning. These protocols should be familiar to all group members so they can support each other when triggers arise.

Michael's triggering experience demonstrates effective trigger management. During his fourth group session, another member shared about his father's alcoholism and violence. Michael suddenly felt transported back to his own childhood, experiencing the same terror and helplessness he'd felt at age eight. He began sweating, his heart raced, and he felt dizzy and nauseous.

The facilitator noticed Michael's distress and offered him a choice: take a break outside the room, stay and use grounding techniques, or continue listening with extra support. Michael chose to stay but moved to a different chair where he felt less trapped and could use bilateral stimulation tools. The facilitator checked in with him periodically while allowing the other member to continue sharing.

After the session, the facilitator briefly processed the experience with Michael, normalizing his response and helping him identify what had been most helpful for staying grounded. This intervention prevented retraumatization while demonstrating that triggers could be managed safely within the group context.

Digital and Hybrid Group Safety Considerations

The COVID-19 pandemic accelerated adoption of digital group therapy platforms, creating new opportunities for accessibility while presenting unique safety challenges. Online and hybrid groups require additional consideration of privacy, technology, and the different dynamics that emerge in virtual spaces. These considerations become particularly important for trauma survivors who may have specific vulnerabilities in digital environments.

Technology privacy extends beyond basic platform security to include helping members understand their own digital safety. This includes using private internet connections rather than public wifi, ensuring family members or roommates cannot overhear sessions, and understanding how to manage their own audio and video settings for comfort and safety.

Physical environment control becomes both easier and more challenging in online formats. Members can participate from their own safe spaces with familiar surroundings and comfort objects, but they also need to ensure privacy and minimize interruptions. Some trauma survivors feel safer in their own environments, while others find the lack of clear boundaries between therapy and home space challenging.

Screen fatigue and dissociation present particular challenges for trauma survivors who may already struggle with dissociation or attention difficulties. Online formats can either support or hinder concentration depending on individual factors. Some members benefit from the option to turn off self-view to reduce self-consciousness, while others need visual contact to stay present and engaged.

Crisis intervention requires different protocols in digital formats, as facilitators cannot provide immediate physical presence or support. Clear crisis plans should include local emergency contacts, safety planning for each member's location, and understanding when online sessions may not be appropriate for individuals in crisis.

Group cohesion may develop differently in virtual formats, requiring intentional strategies to build connection and support between members. This might include structured interaction exercises, breakout room conversations, or creative ways to share and witness each other's experiences across digital barriers.

Hybrid considerations arise when some members attend in person while others participate virtually, creating complex dynamics and potential exclusion of virtual participants. These formats require careful attention to ensuring all members feel equally included and able to participate fully in group process.

Lisa's experience with hybrid participation illustrates these challenges. Due to childcare difficulties and transportation barriers, she joined the group virtually while others attended in person. Initially, she felt like an outsider watching the "real" group through a screen. The facilitator addressed this by ensuring virtual participants were acknowledged first during check-ins, using breakout rooms to pair virtual and in-person members for exercises, and occasionally having everyone participate virtually to equalize the experience.

Building Trust Through Consistency and Attunement

Trust develops slowly for trauma survivors, built through countless small experiences of safety, reliability, and appropriate response to their needs. Group facilitators must demonstrate trustworthiness not just through their actions but through their ability to create and maintain an environment where trust can gradually emerge among group members.

Facilitator consistency includes reliable attendance, predictable responses to group situations, and following through on commitments made to the group. Trauma survivors often test boundaries and commitments, sometimes unconsciously seeking evidence that this relationship will disappoint them like others have. Consistent, appropriate responses help disconfirm these expectations.

Attunement and responsiveness involve recognizing and responding appropriately to both individual and group emotional states. This includes noticing when someone becomes activated and offering support, recognizing when the group energy shifts and adjusting accordingly, and demonstrating that strong emotions can be contained without becoming dangerous or overwhelming.

Transparency about process helps group members understand what's happening and why, reducing anxiety and building trust in the facilitator's competence and intentions. This might include explaining why certain interventions are used, acknowledging when something isn't working well, and being honest about the challenges and limitations of group treatment.

Modeling healthy relationships occurs through facilitator interactions with group members and their responses to group dynamics. Members observe how facilitators handle conflict, express appreciation, maintain boundaries, and recover from mistakes. These observations provide templates for healthy relationship behaviors that many trauma survivors have never experienced.

Cultural humility and responsiveness become essential as group members often come from diverse backgrounds with different experiences of safety, authority, and healing. Facilitators must remain open to learning about cultural factors that influence group members' experiences while avoiding assumptions or stereotypes about different cultural groups.

Robert's trust development illustrates this gradual process. A military veteran with significant authority issues stemming from childhood abuse and military trauma, he initially viewed the group facilitators with suspicion and hostility. He tested boundaries by arriving late, challenging interventions, and making subtly hostile comments about "shrinks who never served."

The facilitators responded with consistency and calm, neither becoming defensive nor attacking Robert's behavior. They acknowledged his military service respectfully, admitted their limitations in understanding combat experience, and maintained clear boundaries about respectful communication while not taking his testing personally.

Over several months, Robert began noticing that these facilitators didn't abuse their authority, didn't punish him for challenging them, and genuinely seemed to care about his wellbeing without trying to control or change him. His testing behaviors gradually decreased as trust developed, and he began participating more authentically in group discussions.

Creating Emotional Holding Environments

The concept of "holding" in therapeutic work refers to the psychological container that allows difficult emotions and experiences to be expressed safely without overwhelming the individual or the group. For trauma survivors, whose emotions may feel dangerous or overwhelming, this holding function becomes essential for therapeutic progress.

Containment skills help group members tolerate strong emotions without becoming flooded or dissociated. These skills might include breathing techniques, grounding exercises, visualization methods, or cognitive strategies for managing overwhelming feelings. Teaching these skills early and practicing them regularly helps build capacity for emotional processing.

Emotional validation provides the acceptance and understanding that many trauma survivors never received for their emotional experiences. This includes acknowledging that their reactions make sense given their experiences, that their emotions are valid and important information, and that they don't need to justify or minimize their feelings.

Normalization of trauma responses helps reduce shame and self-criticism that often accompany trauma symptoms. When group members understand that their responses represent normal adaptations to abnormal circumstances, they can begin developing compassion for themselves and their survival strategies.

Graduated exposure to emotional intensity allows group members to build tolerance gradually rather than becoming overwhelmed by too much too quickly. This might involve starting with less charged topics and gradually approaching more difficult material as group safety and individual capacity develop.

Collective witness provides the powerful experience of having one's pain seen and acknowledged by others who understand. This witnessing goes beyond individual therapy to include the healing that comes from community recognition and support of one's struggles and survival.

Integration support helps group members make meaning of their experiences and connect past trauma to current patterns without becoming stuck in victim identity. This includes recognizing strengths and resilience that enabled survival while working toward post-traumatic growth and thriving.

Addressing Group Dynamics and Process

Group dynamics inevitably emerge as members interact over time, recreating familiar patterns from their families of origin and other significant relationships. These dynamics can either support or interfere with healing, depending on how they are recognized and addressed within the group process.

Scapegoating patterns may emerge when group members unconsciously designate one person to carry difficult emotions or behaviors for the entire group. This pattern often replicates family dynamics where one child was blamed for family problems. Skilled facilitation helps the group recognize these patterns and explore what they might represent for individual members.

Rescuing and caretaking behaviors frequently appear in trauma groups as members attempt to help or fix each other. While the intention is caring, these behaviors can interfere with individual members' need to develop their own coping skills and agency. Groups need to learn the difference between support and enabling.

Competition and jealousy around facilitator attention or group status may activate among members who experienced scarcity of care or attention in their families. These dynamics provide opportunities to work through sibling-like rivalry while learning to celebrate others' progress rather than feeling threatened by it.

Intimacy and distance patterns reflect members' comfort levels with closeness and vulnerability. Some members may push for inappropriate intimacy while others maintain rigid distance. The group provides a laboratory for experimenting with healthy levels of connection and separateness.

Power struggles may emerge between members or between members and facilitators, often reflecting trauma survivors' complicated relationships with authority and control. These struggles can provide valuable material for exploring power dynamics and developing healthier ways of negotiating needs and boundaries.

Safety as an Ongoing Process

Creating safety in trauma groups is not a one-time achievement but an ongoing process that requires constant attention and refinement. Safety needs may change as group members heal and grow, as new members join, or as different topics and experiences emerge in group discussions.

Regular safety check-ins help monitor how safe group members feel and what might be needed to enhance or maintain safety. These check-ins should occur formally at regular intervals but also informally as facilitators notice changes in group dynamics or individual presentations.

Flexibility and adaptation allow safety protocols to evolve based on group needs and feedback. What works for one group composition may not work for another, and safety strategies may need modification as groups develop and change over time.

Learning from ruptures occurs when safety breaks down or trust gets damaged within the group. Rather than viewing these incidents as failures, they can become opportunities for repair, learning, and strengthening of group bonds when handled skillfully.

Graduation and transitions require careful attention to maintaining safety as group composition changes. New members must be integrated thoughtfully while existing members' safety and trust are protected during these transitions.

Path Forward: Safety as Foundation

Safety and trust form the bedrock upon which all other therapeutic work builds. Without this foundation, trauma survivors cannot risk the vulnerability required for healing, cannot tolerate the emotional intensity of processing traumatic experiences, and cannot engage in the interpersonal learning that makes group therapy uniquely powerful.

Creating this foundation requires skill, patience, and deep respect for trauma survivors' protective mechanisms. It demands understanding of how traumatized nervous systems function, appreciation for cultural factors that influence safety perceptions, and commitment to consistency and authenticity in all interactions.

When safety is established, remarkable transformation becomes possible. Group members begin taking emotional risks, sharing authentic experiences, and supporting each other through difficult healing processes. The group becomes a corrective experience that challenges trauma-based assumptions about relationships while providing the interpersonal learning necessary for lasting recovery.

Foundational Elements

- Physical and psychological safety protocols create environmental conditions that support nervous system regulation and therapeutic engagement
- Thoughtful group composition and screening ensure appropriate member matching while maintaining diversity that enriches learning
- Clear norms and boundaries provide structure and predictability while establishing expectations for respectful interaction
- Trigger management systems help members recognize, contain, and process activation safely when it occurs
- Digital and hybrid formats require additional consideration of privacy, technology, and virtual relationship dynamics
- Trust develops through facilitator consistency, attunement, and modeling of healthy relationship behaviors
- Emotional holding environments allow difficult feelings to be expressed and witnessed safely within the group container

Chapter 6: Cultural Considerations and Historical Trauma

Culture is not simply background decoration in the therapy room—it is the lens through which individuals interpret their experiences, understand healing, and make meaning of their struggles. For trauma survivors from diverse cultural backgrounds, this lens may have been shaped by generations of oppression, discrimination, and collective wounds that extend far beyond individual traumatic experiences. Understanding and addressing these cultural factors becomes essential for creating truly effective and inclusive trauma treatment.

The dominant mental health field has historically been designed by and for white, middle-class individuals, often overlooking the ways that cultural factors influence trauma presentation, help-seeking behaviors, and healing processes. This oversight is not merely an academic concern—it directly impacts treatment effectiveness and can inadvertently retraumatize individuals whose cultural experiences are misunderstood or pathologized.

Cultural Formulation in Group Settings

Cultural formulation provides a framework for understanding how cultural factors influence an individual's experience of distress, help-seeking patterns, and treatment preferences. In group settings, this formulation becomes more complex as multiple cultural perspectives interact, potentially creating both rich learning opportunities and challenging dynamics that require skilled navigation.

Cultural identity encompasses multiple, intersecting dimensions including race, ethnicity, religion, sexual orientation, gender identity, socioeconomic status, immigration status, disability status, and regional background. Each dimension contributes to an individual's worldview and may influence their trauma experiences, symptom expression, and treatment expectations.

The process of **cultural identity development** often becomes complicated by trauma, particularly when the trauma involves discrimination, oppression, or violence based on cultural identity factors. Individuals may struggle with positive identification with cultural groups that have been targets of violence, or they may feel disconnected from cultural communities due to trauma-related shame or isolation.

Cultural explanatory models influence how individuals understand their distress and what interventions they believe will be helpful. Some cultures emphasize spiritual or community-based healing approaches, while others focus on individual psychological change. Understanding these models helps therapists work with rather than against clients' existing beliefs about healing.

Power dynamics related to cultural differences require careful attention in group settings. Members from historically marginalized groups may feel unsafe sharing experiences with members from privileged groups, while individuals from privileged backgrounds may need support recognizing their own cultural perspectives and potential impact on others.

Cultural strengths and resources should be identified and incorporated into treatment rather than focusing solely on cultural factors as sources of additional stress or trauma. Many cultures have sophisticated understanding of trauma and healing that can enhance rather than conflict with therapeutic interventions.

Maria's experience illustrates cultural formulation complexity. A 42-year-old Latina woman who immigrated to the United States as a teenager, Maria experienced childhood sexual abuse in her country of origin and domestic violence in her marriage. Her cultural background emphasized family loyalty, religious faith, and collective rather than individual solutions to problems.

Initially, Maria felt uncomfortable in the mixed cultural group, wondering if others would understand her emphasis on family obligations or judge her religious beliefs. She worried that talking about family problems would be seen as betrayal and that her spiritual coping strategies would be dismissed as primitive or ineffective.

The group facilitator helped Maria and other members explore how their cultural backgrounds influenced their trauma experiences and recovery expectations. This process revealed that several members struggled with balancing individual healing needs with cultural values around family loyalty, creating opportunities for mutual support and problem-solving that honored diverse cultural perspectives.

Historical and Intergenerational Trauma Patterns

Individual trauma experiences often occur within contexts of historical and intergenerational trauma that affect entire communities across generations. Understanding these broader trauma patterns helps contextualize individual symptoms while recognizing the collective nature of many traumatic experiences.

Historical trauma refers to the cumulative emotional and psychological wounds transmitted across generations, including the unresolved grief that accompanies these wounds. Native American communities, African American communities, Holocaust survivors and their descendants, refugees from war-torn countries, and other groups have experienced collective traumas that continue affecting community members generations later.

The effects of historical trauma may include higher rates of depression, anxiety, substance abuse, and suicide within affected communities. These patterns reflect not individual pathology but normal responses to abnormal collective experiences that have not been adequately acknowledged or addressed.

Intergenerational transmission occurs through multiple pathways including parenting behaviors, family narratives, epigenetic changes, and community norms that developed as adaptations to historical trauma. Children may absorb their parents' unexpressed grief, fear, or rage without understanding its origins, leading to symptoms that seem disproportionate to their individual experiences.

Cultural trauma emerges when communities experience events that threaten their fundamental assumptions about safety, meaning, and identity. The trauma becomes embedded in cultural memory and continues influencing community members' worldviews and behaviors long after the original events.

Survivor guilt and legacy burdens may affect individuals from historically traumatized communities who achieve success or healing. They may struggle with feeling obligated to carry their ancestors' pain or guilty about moving beyond community patterns of suffering.

Resilience factors often develop within historically traumatized communities, including spiritual practices, community support networks, cultural traditions that promote healing, and collective meaning-making processes that help community members survive and thrive despite ongoing challenges.

James's story demonstrates intergenerational trauma complexity. A 35-year-old African American man whose grandparents migrated north during the Great Migration, James experienced individual trauma through childhood emotional neglect and adult experiences of racial discrimination. However, his symptoms also reflected intergenerational patterns of hypervigilance, emotional restriction, and mistrust of authority that helped his ancestors survive slavery and Jim Crow laws.

In group therapy, James initially struggled to understand why he felt so anxious and angry even when his current life circumstances were relatively stable. Exploring his family history revealed patterns of emotional shutdown and hypervigilance that made sense as survival strategies for previous generations but interfered with his ability to connect with his wife and children.

The group helped James recognize that his symptoms reflected not personal weakness but inherited survival wisdom that no longer served his current circumstances. This reframe reduced his shame while opening possibilities for honoring his ancestors' strength while developing new coping strategies more appropriate to his current life.

Microaggressions and Group Dynamics

Microaggressions—subtle, often unconscious expressions of bias that communicate hostility or derogation toward members of marginalized groups—frequently occur in group settings and can significantly impact safety and therapeutic progress for affected individuals. Understanding and addressing these dynamics becomes essential for inclusive group treatment.

Types of microaggressions include microassaults (conscious, deliberate discriminatory actions), microinsults (unconscious behaviors that convey rudeness or insensitivity), and microinvalidations (communications that exclude or negate the experiences of marginalized individuals). All three types can occur in therapy groups and require different intervention approaches.

Cumulative impact of microaggressions often creates more distress than individual incidents might suggest. For individuals who experience daily microaggressions in their work, school, and community environments, the therapy group may represent one of the few spaces where they hope to find respite from these experiences.

Intersectionality complicates microaggression experiences as individuals with multiple marginalized identities may face complex forms of bias that don't fit simple categories. A Latina lesbian, for example, may experience microaggressions related to both ethnicity and sexual orientation that interact in ways that are difficult to identify or address.

Perpetrator impacts include the reality that well-meaning group members may inadvertently commit microaggressions while genuinely trying to be supportive. These incidents create opportunities for learning and growth but require skilled facilitation to prevent shame and defensive responses that interfere with the therapeutic process.

Bystander dynamics emerge when microaggressions occur and other group members witness but don't intervene. These dynamics can either compound the harm through silence or create opportunities for allyship and support when bystanders respond appropriately.

Therapeutic processing of microaggressions requires balancing validation of affected individuals' experiences with education and growth opportunities for all group members. This processing should avoid placing burden on affected individuals to educate others while ensuring that incidents don't get minimized or ignored.

Sarah's experience with microaggressions illustrates these dynamics. The only person of color in a trauma group composed primarily of white women, Sarah frequently experienced subtle invalidations of her experiences with racism and discrimination. When she shared about job-related stress, other members would minimize her concerns by suggesting that "everyone deals with difficult bosses" without acknowledging the racial dynamics she described.

Initially, Sarah withdrew from group participation, feeling that her experiences weren't understood or valued. The group facilitator noticed this pattern and created space for discussing how different forms of oppression might affect group members' trauma experiences. This conversation revealed that several members had experienced discrimination based on sexual orientation, socioeconomic status, or disability, creating opportunities for mutual understanding and support.

Culturally Adapted Interventions and Screening Tools

Standard trauma assessment tools and therapeutic interventions may not adequately capture or address the experiences of individuals from diverse cultural backgrounds. Culturally adapted approaches improve both assessment accuracy and treatment effectiveness while demonstrating respect for clients' cultural perspectives and values.

Assessment considerations include understanding how different cultures express emotional distress, what symptoms are considered normal versus pathological within specific cultural contexts, and how cultural factors might influence willingness to disclose certain types of experiences or symptoms.

Some cultures emphasize somatic expressions of distress over emotional symptoms, leading to presentations that might be misunderstood or misdiagnosed without cultural awareness. Others may view certain trauma responses as spiritual or supernatural experiences rather than psychological symptoms, requiring different assessment and intervention approaches.

Language factors affect assessment and treatment even when individuals are fluent in English. Trauma experiences may be encoded in native languages, making it difficult to access or process these experiences in English-language therapy. Additionally, concepts like "depression" or "anxiety" may not translate directly across languages, requiring more culturally specific descriptions of internal experiences.

Culturally adapted screening tools have been developed for various populations, including measures that assess historical trauma, discrimination experiences, acculturation stress, and culture-specific expressions of distress. These tools provide more accurate assessment while demonstrating cultural responsiveness.

Intervention adaptations might include incorporating cultural healing practices, involving family or community members appropriately, addressing culture-specific aspects of trauma experiences, and modifying standard interventions to align with cultural values and beliefs.

Spiritual and religious considerations require understanding how individuals' faith traditions influence their understanding of trauma, healing, and therapeutic change. Some interventions may conflict with religious beliefs, while others can be enhanced through incorporation of appropriate spiritual practices.

Community involvement may be essential for individuals from cultures that emphasize collective rather than individual approaches to healing. This might include involving extended family members, religious leaders, or community elders in appropriate ways while maintaining therapeutic boundaries and confidentiality.

Roberto's treatment illustrates culturally adapted intervention needs. A recent immigrant from El Salvador who experienced both war trauma in his country of origin and discrimination stress in the United States, Roberto initially struggled with standard PTSD assessment tools that didn't capture his complex trauma experiences.

His symptoms included what he described as "susto" (soul loss), a culturally recognized condition that involves feeling like part of his spirit remained trapped in traumatic experiences. Standard depression and anxiety measures didn't adequately capture this spiritual dimension of his distress, leading to incomplete assessment and treatment planning.

The therapist worked with Roberto to understand his cultural explanatory model for his distress and incorporated appropriate healing practices including prayer, connection with his cultural community, and interventions that addressed the spiritual as well as psychological aspects of his trauma. This approach honored his cultural perspective while providing effective trauma treatment.

Working with Diverse Populations and Belief Systems

Group therapy brings together individuals with different cultural backgrounds, belief systems, and worldviews, creating both opportunities for learning and challenges around managing differences respectfully. Successful multicultural groups require skilled facilitation that honors diversity while building connections across differences.

Religious and spiritual diversity may include members from different faith traditions, individuals who have been harmed by religious institutions, those who find spiritual practices essential to healing, and others who prefer secular approaches. Managing these differences requires creating space for all perspectives while ensuring that no one feels pressured to adopt beliefs that conflict with their own values.

Socioeconomic differences can create significant dynamics within groups as members may have vastly different experiences with financial stress, educational opportunities, housing stability, and access to resources. These differences can trigger shame, envy, or judgment if not addressed thoughtfully.

Sexual orientation and gender identity diversity requires creating inclusive environments where LGBTQ+ individuals feel safe to be authentic while also ensuring that members from more conservative backgrounds feel comfortable participating. This balance requires ongoing attention to language, assumptions, and group norms.

Generational differences may emerge between older and younger group members who have different cultural experiences, communication styles, and perspectives on healing and change. These differences can create learning opportunities when managed skillfully.

Immigration and acculturation issues affect many group members who may be navigating complex cultural identities while dealing with trauma experiences. First-generation immigrants may struggle with different issues than second or third-generation individuals, requiring understanding of acculturation processes and their relationship to trauma and healing.

Disability and neurodiversity considerations ensure that group processes accommodate different learning styles, communication needs, and accessibility requirements while fostering understanding about how disability experiences intersect with trauma.

The multicultural trauma group that included David illustrates these dynamics. Group members included a Native American veteran, an African American woman who experienced childhood abuse, a white gay male survivor of hate crimes, a Latina immigrant with domestic violence history, and an older white woman with medical trauma experiences.

Initially, members struggled to find common ground across their different experiences and backgrounds. The Native American veteran felt that others couldn't understand the particular forms of historical and cultural trauma affecting his community. The gay member worried that the older woman would judge his lifestyle. The immigrant feared that others would blame her for staying in an abusive relationship.

Through skilled facilitation, the group gradually recognized both their differences and their shared experiences of trauma, resilience, and the search for healing. Members learned from each other's perspectives while finding universal themes of survival, strength, and hope that connected them across cultural differences.

Addressing Systemic Oppression and Social Justice

Individual trauma often occurs within contexts of systemic oppression and social injustice that continue affecting individuals' daily lives even during treatment. Effective culturally responsive trauma therapy must address these systemic factors rather than focusing solely on individual symptoms and coping strategies.

Discrimination and oppression as ongoing stressors require acknowledgment and intervention in trauma treatment. Individuals who experience daily racism, homophobia, transphobia, or other forms of discrimination may struggle to recover from historical trauma while continuing to experience current trauma through oppression.

Social justice healing recognizes that individual healing may be incomplete without addressing systemic factors that contribute to trauma and interfere with recovery. This might include advocacy, community organizing, or collective action as components of healing process.

Empowerment approaches help individuals recognize their strengths and agency while working to change systems that perpetuate trauma and oppression. These approaches balance individual therapy with social action and community involvement.

Ally development among group members from privileged backgrounds can create opportunities for mutual support and systemic change. Members with privilege can learn to use their advantages to support marginalized community members while understanding their own roles in systemic oppression.

Trauma-informed social justice recognizes that many social justice advocates have trauma histories that may influence their activism while understanding that engagement in social change can be healing for trauma survivors who feel empowered to create positive change.

Institutional responses may be necessary when trauma treatment organizations perpetuate systemic oppression through their policies, practices, or staff behaviors. Addressing these institutional factors becomes essential for creating truly culturally responsive treatment environments.

Integration and Healing Across Cultures

Successful multicultural trauma groups create environments where healing occurs both through connection across differences and through affirmation of individual cultural identities. This integration requires ongoing attention to both individual and collective needs while fostering environments of mutual respect and understanding.

Cultural pride and identity affirmation help group members develop positive connections to their cultural backgrounds while processing trauma experiences that may have created shame or disconnection from cultural communities. Healing often involves reclaiming cultural strengths and resources that trauma may have obscured.

Bicultural competence develops as individuals learn to navigate multiple cultural contexts while maintaining authentic connections to their various cultural identities. This skill becomes particularly important for individuals from marginalized communities who must function in dominant culture environments.

Collective healing emerges when group members recognize shared experiences of oppression, resilience, and recovery across different cultural backgrounds. This recognition creates solidarity and mutual support that extends beyond individual healing to community and societal change.

Cultural bridging occurs when group members learn from each other's cultural perspectives and healing practices, creating hybrid approaches that draw from multiple traditions while respecting the integrity of each cultural framework.

Moving Forward with Cultural Wisdom

Cultural considerations in trauma group treatment are not add-on features or special accommodations—they are fundamental aspects of effective, ethical treatment that honors the full humanity and complexity of trauma survivors' experiences. Understanding and integrating cultural factors requires ongoing learning, humility, and commitment to creating inclusive healing environments.

The goal is not cultural colorblindness that ignores important differences but cultural responsiveness that honors both diversity and common human experiences of trauma and healing. When achieved skillfully, multicultural trauma groups become powerful environments for both individual recovery and social healing that extends beyond the therapy room to communities and societies.

Wisdom for Practice

- Cultural formulation provides frameworks for understanding how multiple cultural identities influence trauma experiences and treatment expectations
- Historical and intergenerational trauma patterns contextualize individual symptoms within broader collective experiences of oppression and resilience

- Microaggressions in group settings require skilled recognition and intervention to maintain safety for marginalized group members
- Culturally adapted screening tools and interventions improve assessment accuracy and treatment effectiveness across diverse populations
- Managing religious, socioeconomic, and other forms of diversity requires creating inclusive environments that honor different perspectives
- Addressing systemic oppression and social justice factors becomes essential for comprehensive trauma treatment
- Integration and healing across cultures creates opportunities for both individual recovery and collective transformation

Chapter 7: Group Formation and Psychoeducation (Sessions 1-3)

The first three sessions of trauma group therapy carry immense weight—they determine if strangers will become allies in healing or if the group will dissolve before it truly begins. These early meetings are not simply administrative sessions but carefully orchestrated experiences that lay the groundwork for everything that follows. You're creating the foundation upon which traumatized individuals will risk vulnerability, challenge their deepest beliefs about relationships, and practice new ways of being with others.

Think of these initial sessions as planting seeds in soil that may have been barren for years. The ground must be prepared carefully, nutrients added gradually, and conditions optimized before any growth can occur. Rush this process, and the seeds won't take root. Provide insufficient care, and they'll wither before sprouting. But create the right conditions, and remarkable transformation becomes possible.

Pre-group Preparation and Individual Meetings

The work begins long before group members sit together for the first time. Individual preparation meetings serve multiple functions: they assess readiness, begin psychoeducation, establish therapeutic rapport, and reduce anxiety about group participation. These meetings can make the difference between successful group integration and premature dropout.

Assessment of readiness goes beyond standard screening criteria to understand each individual's unique presentation, triggers, and capacity for group participation. You're looking for both red flags that might indicate contraindications and green lights that suggest group therapy will be beneficial. This assessment includes current symptom severity, interpersonal functioning, motivation for change, and realistic expectations about group process.

Psychoeducation introduction begins during individual meetings, providing basic information about trauma, its effects on the nervous system, and how group therapy works. This early education reduces anxiety while establishing you as a knowledgeable, trustworthy guide. Many trauma survivors have been misunderstood or pathologized by mental health professionals, so demonstrating competence and understanding becomes crucial for engagement.

Rapport building occurs through these individual contacts, allowing potential group members to experience your therapeutic style and decide if they feel safe enough to participate. Some individuals need multiple individual meetings before feeling ready for group participation, and this additional time often pays dividends in terms of group engagement and retention.

Anxiety reduction happens naturally when individuals know what to expect, understand the group structure, and feel prepared for their first group experience. You can address specific concerns, answer questions, and provide coping strategies for managing group-related anxiety.

Consider Maria's preparation process. A 34-year-old survivor of childhood sexual abuse and domestic violence, she initially felt terrified about sharing her experiences with strangers. During her individual preparation meetings, she expressed fears that others would judge her for staying in an abusive marriage or blame her for the childhood abuse. She worried that hearing others' stories would trigger her own memories and that she might dissociate during group sessions.

The therapist spent two individual sessions helping Maria understand trauma responses, normalize her concerns, and develop coping strategies for group participation. They practiced grounding techniques, discussed what to do if she became triggered, and established signals she could use to communicate her needs during group sessions. By the time Maria attended her first group meeting, she felt anxious but prepared—a manageable combination that allowed for successful engagement.

Logistical preparation includes practical details about group meeting times, location, what to bring, and how to handle unexpected absence or lateness. These details matter enormously to trauma survivors who often cope through control and predictability. Providing clear, written information reduces anxiety while demonstrating reliability and organization.

Goal setting begins during individual meetings as you help potential members identify what they hope to gain from group participation. These goals provide direction for group work while establishing realistic expectations about the change process. Goals should be specific, measurable, and achievable within the group timeframe.

Robert's goal-setting process illustrates this preparation phase. A 42-year-old combat veteran struggling with anger, isolation, and relationship difficulties, Robert initially expressed skepticism about group therapy's potential benefits. He'd tried individual therapy multiple times with limited success and viewed groups as "touchy-feely BS that won't work for someone like me."

During preparation meetings, the therapist helped Robert identify specific, practical goals that aligned with his values and concerns. Rather than vague goals like "feel better," Robert established concrete objectives: improve communication with his wife, reduce explosive anger episodes, develop friendships with other veterans, and sleep better at night. These tangible goals provided motivation for group participation while establishing criteria for measuring progress.

Trauma Psychoeducation Using Current Neuroscience

The first group session should provide a solid foundation of trauma education that helps members understand their experiences through a scientific, non-pathologizing lens. This education reduces shame, provides hope, and establishes common language for group discussions. Modern neuroscience offers powerful explanations for trauma responses that help survivors understand they're not "broken" but rather experiencing normal reactions to abnormal events.

Brain basics provide the foundation for trauma education, explaining how the brain develops, functions, and responds to threat. You don't need extensive neuroanatomy, but basic understanding of the amygdala, hippocampus, and prefrontal cortex helps group members understand their experiences. Use simple analogies—the amygdala as smoke detector, the prefrontal cortex as CEO—to make complex concepts accessible.

Trauma's impact on the brain explains how overwhelming experiences affect neural development and functioning. Chronic trauma exposure changes brain structure and function, creating the symptoms that bring people to treatment. This biological explanation reduces self-blame while providing hope that brains can heal and change throughout life.

The nervous system response introduces concepts from polyvagal theory in accessible language. Group members learn about fight, flight, freeze, and fawn responses as adaptive survival strategies rather than personal failures. This education helps normalize their reactions while providing frameworks for understanding current symptoms.

Trauma types and their effects help group members understand different categories of trauma and their unique impacts. This includes developmental versus adult trauma, single-incident versus complex trauma, and interpersonal versus impersonal trauma. Understanding these distinctions helps members recognize their own experiences while appreciating others' different presentations.

The window of tolerance provides a visual framework for understanding emotional regulation challenges. Group members learn to identify their own windows and recognize when they're in hyperarousal or hypoarousal states. This concept becomes a cornerstone for all future group work as members learn to monitor and manage their nervous system states.

During the first session of Jennifer's group, the therapist used a simple drawing to illustrate trauma's impact on the brain. She drew three circles representing the amygdala, hippocampus, and prefrontal cortex, explaining how trauma affects each region. Jennifer later reported that this explanation helped her understand why she couldn't "just get over" her childhood abuse and why her reactions sometimes seemed disproportionate to current situations.

The therapist explained how Jennifer's amygdala had become hyperactive due to repeated childhood threats, creating the hypervigilance and anxiety she experienced daily. Her hippocampus had been affected by chronic stress hormones, making it difficult to distinguish between past and present threats. Her prefrontal cortex sometimes went "offline" during stress, explaining why she felt out of control during triggered states.

This education didn't eliminate Jennifer's symptoms, but it provided a framework for understanding them that reduced shame and self-criticism. She began recognizing triggered states as biological responses rather than personal failures, creating space for self-compassion and more effective coping strategies.

Introduction to Schema Concepts and Mode Mapping

Schema therapy concepts provide another layer of psychoeducation that helps group members understand their patterns of thinking, feeling, and behaving. Introducing schemas and modes early creates common language for group discussions while providing frameworks for understanding interpersonal dynamics as they emerge.

Early maladaptive schemas represent core beliefs about self and others that develop during childhood and persist throughout life. These beliefs make sense given traumatic experiences but often interfere with adult functioning and relationships. Introducing schema concepts helps group members recognize their own patterns while understanding others' responses.

Schema domains organize the 18 early maladaptive schemas into five categories that represent different areas of psychological need: disconnection and rejection, impaired autonomy and performance, impaired limits, other-directedness, and overvigilance and inhibition.

Understanding these domains helps group members identify their core areas of difficulty.

Schema modes represent emotional and behavioral states that emerge in response to various triggers and situations. Modes provide a framework for understanding the different "parts" of personality that trauma survivors often experience. This concept helps normalize the internal conflicts and rapid emotional shifts that characterize complex trauma.

Child modes include the vulnerable child (containing core emotional pain), angry child (expressing natural protest against unfair treatment), and impulsive child (seeking immediate gratification or relief). These modes represent different aspects of the authentic self that were affected by trauma.

Parent modes include the punitive parent (internalized critical voices) and demanding parent (impossibly high standards and expectations). These modes often sound like harsh caregivers from childhood and create internal criticism and pressure that interfere with healing.

Coping modes represent protective strategies that help manage schema activation but often create their own problems. These include the detached protector (emotional withdrawal), compliant surrenderer (giving up personal needs), and self-aggrandizer (false superiority to defend against vulnerability).

The healthy adult mode represents the integrated, functional aspect of personality that can respond flexibly to situations while caring for wounded parts. Developing this mode becomes a central focus of schema therapy work.

During the second session, Michael's group engaged in a mode identification exercise. Group members received descriptions of different modes and identified which ones felt familiar to them. Michael immediately recognized the detached protector mode—his tendency to withdraw emotionally when relationships became too intense or demanding.

77

He also identified with the punitive parent mode, recognizing the harsh internal voice that constantly criticized his performance and told him he was weak for needing help. The vulnerable child mode felt more difficult to acknowledge, but he could identify the scared, hurt part of him that rarely felt safe enough to emerge.

This exercise created immediate connections between group members as they recognized shared patterns across different life experiences. Sarah identified with Michael's detached protector mode, while Robert related to his angry child mode. These connections began building group cohesion while providing language for discussing internal experiences.

Group Rules, Confidentiality, and Crisis Protocols

Clear structure and safety protocols provide the container necessary for trauma processing. These agreements must be established early and reinforced consistently to create the predictability and safety that trauma survivors need for healing. The rules should be practical, enforceable, and designed to protect both individual members and group integrity.

Confidentiality agreements form the foundation of group safety. Members must understand that what's shared in group stays in group, with clear exceptions for safety concerns. This includes not discussing other members' information outside of group, avoiding social media connections with group members, and understanding the limits of confidentiality regarding safety issues.

Attendance expectations balance the need for commitment with recognition that trauma survivors may struggle with consistency. Reasonable expectations might include attending at least 75% of sessions, notifying the group about planned absences, and discussing attendance problems openly rather than simply disappearing.

Communication guidelines establish how group members will interact respectfully during emotionally charged discussions. These include speaking directly to each other rather than through the facilitator, using "I" statements to express reactions, avoiding advice-giving unless requested, and respecting others' right to their experiences.

Physical safety protocols address trauma survivors' often-complicated relationships with touch and personal space. Clear agreements about no uninvited physical contact, respecting personal space preferences, and asking permission before offering comfort help prevent inadvertent triggering.

Crisis protocols outline what happens when group members become severely distressed, dissociate, or express suicidal thoughts during sessions. These protocols should include immediate safety assessment, available resources, and clear procedures for handling psychiatric emergencies.

Between-session contact guidelines clarify how group members can support each other outside of sessions while maintaining appropriate boundaries. This might include exchanging phone numbers for crisis support while avoiding lengthy phone conversations that could interfere with group process.

Lisa's group spent considerable time during the third session establishing crisis protocols after she disclosed previous suicide attempts. The group developed clear agreements about how to respond if someone expressed suicidal thoughts during sessions, including immediate safety assessment, developing safety plans, and appropriate follow-up procedures.

They also discussed between-session support, establishing that group members could contact each other for brief check-ins during difficult times but should avoid lengthy conversations about trauma material outside of group sessions. These agreements provided structure while respecting both individual needs and group boundaries.

Early Bonding Exercises and Safety Building

The first three sessions must balance psychoeducation with relationship building to create group cohesion and safety. Early bonding exercises help members begin connecting with each other while respecting their comfort levels and protective mechanisms. These exercises should be structured, optional, and designed to promote safety rather than premature vulnerability.

Name and intention sharing provides a simple way for members to introduce themselves while setting intentions for group participation. This exercise allows for varying levels of disclosure—some members might share extensive background information while others provide only basic introductions. The key is allowing choice while encouraging participation.

Strength identification helps group members recognize positive qualities and resources they bring to the group. This exercise counters the deficit focus that trauma survivors often carry while helping members see each other as resources rather than just sources of problems. Strengths might include survival skills, life experiences, personal qualities, or specific knowledge.

Hope and concern sharing allows members to express both their hopes for group participation and their concerns about the process. This exercise normalizes anxiety while helping members realize they share similar hopes and fears. It also provides valuable information about what members need to feel safe and engaged.

Grounding practice introduces nervous system regulation techniques that will be used throughout the group. Starting with simple breathing exercises or mindfulness practices helps members develop regulation skills while experiencing group co-regulation. These practices become essential tools for managing activation during more intense sessions.

Safety assessment involves checking in about how safe members feel in the group and what might increase their sense of safety. This ongoing process helps identify potential problems early while demonstrating the facilitators' commitment to maintaining safety as the primary concern.

During Robert's group formation, the strength identification exercise proved particularly powerful. Initially reluctant to share positive qualities about himself, Robert was surprised when other group members identified strengths they observed in him—his protective instincts toward others, his loyalty to friends, his resilience in surviving combat experiences.

This feedback challenged Robert's self-perception as a "broken" person and helped him recognize resources he brought to the group. When Jennifer shared that his calm presence made her feel safer, Robert experienced himself as a positive force rather than a burden. This early positive feedback created investment in group success while beginning to challenge his negative self-schema.

The group also practiced simple grounding techniques together, including focused breathing and 5-4-3-2-1 sensory exercises. These shared experiences created connection while providing tools that members could use both during sessions and in their daily lives. The co-regulation that occurred during these exercises gave members a taste of how the group could support their healing.

Building Momentum for Deeper Work

The success of these first three sessions largely determines whether the group will develop into a cohesive, healing community or struggle with attendance, safety concerns, and superficial engagement. By the end of session three, members should feel knowledgeable about trauma and its effects, familiar with basic schema concepts, clear about group expectations, and connected enough with other members to risk deeper sharing.

You'll know you've succeeded when members express both excitement and nervousness about continuing, when they reference things other members have shared, and when they begin using the language you've introduced to describe their experiences. Members should feel hopeful about the possibility of change while realistic about the work required.

The foundation you build during these sessions will be tested repeatedly as the group moves into more challenging territory. Members will trigger each other, old patterns will emerge, and resistance will surface. But if you've created sufficient safety and understanding during formation, the group will have resources to navigate these challenges successfully.

The psychoeducation provided during these sessions shouldn't end here but should continue throughout the group as members develop capacity to understand more complex concepts and integrate new information with their ongoing experiences. The initial education creates scaffolding upon which deeper learning can build.

Stepping Forward Together

These foundational sessions require patience, skill, and trust in the process. You're asking traumatized individuals to risk vulnerability with strangers based on the promise that healing is possible through connection. That's a significant leap of faith that requires careful preparation and gradual trust-building.

The success of group formation often determines the entire group's trajectory. Members who feel safe, informed, and connected during these early sessions are much more likely to engage authentically throughout the group process. Those who feel overwhelmed, confused, or disconnected may dropout before experiencing the group's benefits.

The next phase of group work will test the foundation you've built as members begin identifying their specific schemas and modes. The safety and connection created during formation will be essential resources as members navigate the more challenging territory ahead.

Essential Learning Elements

- Individual preparation meetings assess readiness, begin psychoeducation, and reduce anxiety about group participation

- Trauma psychoeducation using current neuroscience reduces shame while providing frameworks for understanding symptoms
- Schema concepts and mode mapping create common language for discussing internal experiences and interpersonal patterns
- Clear rules, confidentiality agreements, and crisis protocols provide the structure necessary for psychological safety
- Early bonding exercises build connection while respecting members' comfort levels and protective mechanisms
- Successful group formation creates the foundation for all subsequent healing work and largely determines group outcomes

Chapter 8: Schema Identification and Mode Mapping (Sessions 4-6)

The group has found its rhythm—members arrive on time, settle into familiar seats, and exchange brief greetings that suggest growing comfort with each other. But now comes the real work. Sessions four through six mark the transition from general trauma education to personal exploration, from shared learning to individual vulnerability. This is where group members begin mapping the specific patterns that have shaped their lives, often for decades.

You're no longer dealing with abstract concepts but with the lived reality of each person's internal world. The schemas and modes you introduced in earlier sessions now have faces, voices, and personal histories attached to them. Members will recognize themselves in ways that can be both relieving ("I'm not crazy—this makes sense") and overwhelming ("How do I change patterns that feel like who I am?").

Schema Questionnaires and Group Processing

The Young Schema Questionnaire (15) provides a structured entry point into schema identification, offering validated measures of the 18 early maladaptive schemas across five domains. But administering questionnaires in group settings requires careful consideration of how to process results in ways that promote learning while maintaining safety and avoiding comparison competitions.

Pre-session questionnaire completion allows members to reflect privately on their responses before group discussion. This individual processing time reduces anxiety while allowing members to prepare for sharing that feels manageable. Some members may want to complete questionnaires at home, while others prefer the structure of in-session completion with immediate support available.

Scoring and interpretation should be handled sensitively, recognizing that some members may feel overwhelmed by high scores across multiple schemas while others might minimize their difficulties. The focus should be on patterns and themes rather than specific numerical scores, using results as starting points for exploration rather than definitive diagnoses.

Group processing guidelines help create structure for discussing personal schema profiles while maintaining safety and respect. These might include sharing only schemas that feel comfortable to discuss, focusing on current patterns rather than traumatic origins, and avoiding comparisons or judgments about others' profiles.

Normalization and validation occur as members recognize shared schemas across different life experiences. This process reduces isolation while demonstrating that schemas represent understandable adaptations to difficult circumstances rather than personal failings or character defects.

Sarah's schema profile illustrated the complexity of trauma survivors' presentations. Her highest scores appeared on abandonment/instability, mistrust/abuse, emotional deprivation, defectiveness/shame, and vulnerability to harm schemas—a pattern reflecting her childhood experiences of parental neglect and sexual abuse by a family friend.

During group processing, Sarah initially felt overwhelmed by her "high scores," interpreting them as evidence that she was "more damaged" than other members. The facilitator helped reframe these results as information about adaptive strategies Sarah had developed to survive threatening circumstances, emphasizing her resilience rather than her pathology.

When Robert shared that he also scored high on mistrust/abuse and defectiveness schemas despite his very different combat trauma history, Sarah began recognizing universal themes in trauma responses. This normalization reduced her shame while helping her see patterns as changeable rather than fixed personality traits.

Cultural considerations must be addressed when using standardized questionnaires, as some items may not translate well across different cultural backgrounds or may reflect cultural values rather than psychopathology. Group discussion can help distinguish between cultural patterns and trauma-related schemas while respecting diverse perspectives on relationships and emotional expression.

Individual variations in questionnaire responses provide opportunities for learning about different presentations of similar schemas. Some members may score high on schemas but show different behavioral expressions, while others may have similar scores but very different life experiences that created those patterns.

Michael's schema profile showed high scores on emotional deprivation and social isolation despite his successful career and marriage. During group discussion, he explored how these schemas manifested differently than Sarah's—through workaholism and emotional distance rather than obvious relationship difficulties. This comparison helped both members recognize how schemas can be expressed in various ways while serving similar protective functions.

Creating Individual Schema Profiles

Moving beyond questionnaire scores to create individualized schema profiles requires helping group members understand how their specific schemas interact, how they developed, and how they currently influence thoughts, feelings, and behaviors. This process transforms abstract concepts into personal roadmaps for change.

Schema interactions often create complex patterns where multiple schemas reinforce each other. Someone with abandonment and defectiveness schemas might interpret neutral relationship events as evidence of both impending rejection and personal unworthiness. Understanding these interactions helps explain why changing one pattern often requires addressing several schemas simultaneously.

Historical development connects current schemas to past experiences without requiring detailed trauma processing at this stage. Members can begin recognizing how their schemas made sense given their childhood circumstances while understanding that adaptive strategies may no longer serve them effectively.

Current manifestations help members recognize how schemas influence their daily lives through specific thoughts, emotions, and behaviors. This awareness creates possibilities for change by highlighting automatic patterns that previously operated outside conscious recognition.

Triggers and activation identify specific situations, people, or events that tend to activate particular schemas. Understanding these triggers provides early warning systems that can help members recognize schema activation before it leads to problematic responses.

Protective strategies help members recognize the coping mechanisms they've developed to manage schema activation. These strategies often include the modes introduced earlier—detached protector, compliant surrenderer, or self-aggrandizer—and understanding them reduces self-criticism while highlighting both adaptive and maladaptive aspects.

Jennifer's schema profile revealed strong abandonment, mistrust, and defectiveness patterns stemming from childhood emotional abuse and neglect. Through group discussion, she began recognizing how these schemas interacted to create her relationship patterns—choosing emotionally unavailable partners (confirming abandonment expectations), becoming hypervigilant for signs of rejection (mistrust activation), and interpreting partners' normal needs for space as evidence of her inadequacy (defectiveness confirmation).

Her schema triggers included partners being late, forgetting plans, or spending time with friends without her. When activated, Jennifer's typical response involved the compliant surrenderer mode—becoming overly accommodating while suppressing her own needs to prevent abandonment. This pattern had protected her from overt rejection but left her feeling resentful and emotionally depleted.

Understanding these patterns helped Jennifer recognize that her responses made perfect sense given her childhood experiences of emotional abandonment and criticism. This awareness reduced self-blame while creating possibilities for developing new responses that honored both her protective needs and her desires for authentic connection.

Mode Identification Through Experiential Exercises

While questionnaires provide valuable information about schemas, modes often become more apparent through experiential exercises that access emotional and somatic responses. These exercises help group members recognize their different internal states while providing direct experience of mode shifts and their effects.

Body awareness exercises help members notice physical sensations associated with different modes. The vulnerable child mode might create tightness in the chest or throat, while the detached protector mode could manifest as numbness or disconnection from bodily sensations. Developing this somatic awareness provides early warning systems for mode activation.

Voice and posture changes often accompany mode shifts, and helping members notice these changes increases awareness while providing information about internal states to both individuals and group members. The punitive parent mode might create rigid posture and harsh vocal tones, while the vulnerable child mode could manifest through softer speech and protective body positions.

Imagery and visualization exercises can help members access different modes safely while maintaining present-moment awareness. These might include visualizing younger versions of themselves, imagining conversations with critical internal voices, or creating safe spaces for vulnerable parts to emerge and be witnessed.

Role-playing exercises allow members to experiment with expressing different modes while receiving feedback from group members. These exercises should be carefully structured to maintain safety while providing opportunities for authentic expression and validation.

Mode dialogues help members recognize internal conflicts between different modes while developing the healthy adult's capacity to mediate these conflicts. Members might practice conversations between their vulnerable child and punitive parent modes, with support from group members and facilitators.

During a body awareness exercise in David's group, members were guided through a meditation focusing on physical sensations while thinking about recent stressful events. David noticed that thinking about conflict with his supervisor created immediate tension in his shoulders and jaw, along with a sense of his body becoming smaller and more protected.

The facilitator helped David recognize this as his vulnerable child mode—the scared, powerless feelings he'd experienced as a child when his father would criticize and yell at him. In contrast, when David imagined standing up to his supervisor, his posture straightened, his jaw set firmly, and his voice became harder. This represented his angry child mode, rarely expressed but carrying decades of suppressed rage about unfair treatment.

Through group feedback, David learned that other members could observe these mode shifts through changes in his facial expression, posture, and vocal tone. This external validation helped him trust his internal awareness while recognizing that modes were visible aspects of his personality rather than hidden psychological problems.

Group Feedback and Validation Processes

Structured feedback processes help group members learn about their schemas and modes through others' observations while building interpersonal skills and group cohesion. This feedback should be offered carefully to avoid triggering defensive responses while providing valuable information about interpersonal impact.

Feedback guidelines ensure that observations are offered respectfully and received openly. These might include focusing on specific behaviors rather than general personality traits, using "I" statements to express personal reactions, balancing challenging observations with supportive comments, and checking for consent before offering potentially difficult feedback.

Validation practices help members feel seen and understood in their schema presentations rather than judged or criticized. Validation involves acknowledging that schemas and modes make sense given individual histories while expressing appreciation for members' courage in sharing vulnerable aspects of themselves.

Pattern recognition occurs as group members observe similarities and differences in how schemas manifest across different individuals. These observations help normalize schema presentations while highlighting unique aspects of each person's adaptive strategies.

Interpersonal impact feedback helps members understand how their schemas and modes affect others, providing valuable information about relationship patterns that may operate outside their awareness. This feedback should be offered gently and received as information rather than criticism.

Strength identification balances feedback about challenging patterns with recognition of positive qualities, adaptive strategies, and resources that members demonstrate. Even problematic modes often contain valuable aspects that can be honored while working toward more flexible responses.

Lisa received particularly valuable feedback about her compliant surrenderer mode during the sixth session. Group members had observed her tendency to defer to others' opinions, apologize frequently, and minimize her own needs during group discussions. Initially, Lisa felt criticized and defensive, interpreting the feedback as confirmation of her defectiveness schema.

The facilitator helped reframe this feedback as information about protective strategies that had helped Lisa survive childhood abuse but might limit her ability to develop authentic relationships. Group members shared their appreciation for Lisa's caring nature and sensitivity to others' needs while expressing concern that she might not be getting her own needs met.

Robert shared that Lisa's tendency to defer reminded him of his own wife's people-pleasing patterns, helping him recognize how these behaviors affected partners. Jennifer expressed appreciation for Lisa's gentleness while encouraging her to share her own opinions more directly. This balanced feedback helped Lisa begin recognizing her impact on others while feeling supported rather than criticized.

Developing Mode Awareness Between Sessions

Schema and mode work cannot be limited to group sessions if lasting change is to occur. Members need tools and strategies for recognizing schema activation and mode shifts in their daily lives while practicing new responses outside the safety of the group environment.

Daily awareness practices help members notice schema triggers and mode shifts as they occur in real-life situations. These might include brief check-ins with internal states throughout the day, keeping journals about schema activation episodes, or using smartphone apps to track mood and trigger patterns.

Mode monitoring involves developing awareness of when different modes become active and what triggers these shifts. Members can learn to recognize early warning signs of mode activation while developing strategies for responding more consciously to triggering situations.

Healthy adult development requires practicing the integrated, flexible responses that characterize mature functioning. This might involve challenging punitive parent messages, nurturing vulnerable child parts, or setting appropriate limits with compliant surrenderer tendencies.

Support system utilization helps members identify people in their lives who can provide validation and reality-checking when schemas become activated. This might include family members, friends, or other group members who can offer perspective during difficult times.

Homework assignments provide structured opportunities for practicing new awareness and responses between sessions. These assignments should be specific, achievable, and designed to build on group learning while promoting real-world application.

Michael developed a daily practice of checking in with his internal state three times per day—morning, midday, and evening—using his phone to set reminder alarms. During these brief check-ins, he would notice his current mode, identify any triggers that had activated schemas, and practice brief grounding exercises if needed.

He also created a simple rating system for schema activation intensity, tracking patterns over time to identify high-risk situations and effective coping strategies. This data helped him recognize that work conflicts consistently triggered his defectiveness and failure schemas, while time with his children activated more positive states.

Between sessions, Michael practiced recognizing his detached protector mode when it emerged during emotionally charged conversations with his wife. Instead of automatically withdrawing, he began experimenting with staying present and expressing his needs more directly. These experiments provided valuable material for group discussion while building confidence in his ability to change established patterns.

Integration and Preparation for Deeper Work

Sessions four through six represent a turning point in group process as members move from learning about trauma and schemas in general to recognizing their specific patterns and beginning to change them. This transition can feel overwhelming as the work becomes more personal and the possibility of change feels both exciting and terrifying.

Success indicators at this stage include members using schema and mode language to describe their experiences, recognizing patterns that previously operated outside awareness, expressing curiosity about change possibilities, and beginning to challenge automatic responses in small ways.

Common challenges might include feeling overwhelmed by the extent of schema patterns, comparing themselves negatively to other group members, experiencing increased symptoms as awareness grows, or feeling hopeless about the possibility of changing long-standing patterns.

Resistance and ambivalence are normal responses as members recognize how much of their identity has been organized around schema patterns. Change can feel threatening even when current patterns create problems, as familiar responses provide predictability and perceived safety.

Group cohesion building continues as members share increasingly personal information and provide mutual support during schema exploration. The bonds formed during this phase often sustain members through more challenging phases of group work.

Preparation for trauma processing begins as members develop greater awareness of their internal states and coping resources. The self-awareness and regulation skills developed during schema identification provide essential foundations for the trauma processing work that follows.

The group's transformation during these sessions can be remarkable to witness. Members who arrived feeling broken and alone begin recognizing that their responses make sense, that others share similar struggles, and that change is possible with support and practice. The shame that often accompanies trauma symptoms begins dissolving in the light of understanding and acceptance.

Building on Understanding

These sessions create the roadmap that will guide the remainder of group work. Members now understand their specific patterns, recognize how these patterns developed, and have begun imagining different ways of responding to life's challenges. But understanding alone doesn't create change—that requires the experiential work that lies ahead.

The schemas and modes identified during these sessions will appear repeatedly throughout the remaining group work, providing frameworks for understanding reactions, processing traumatic experiences, and practicing new responses. This foundational work makes everything that follows more meaningful and effective.

Core Learning Points

- Schema questionnaires provide structured entry points for identifying personal patterns while requiring careful processing to maintain safety
- Individual schema profiles help members understand how multiple schemas interact and influence daily life experiences
- Experiential exercises access emotional and somatic responses that reveal mode presentations more clearly than questionnaires alone
- Structured group feedback processes provide valuable interpersonal learning while building validation and support skills
- Between-session awareness practices help members recognize schema activation in daily life while practicing new responses
- These sessions create essential foundations for trauma processing by developing self-awareness and internal monitoring capabilities

Chapter 9: Neurobiology and Somatic Interventions (Sessions 7-9)

The body holds what the mind cannot yet process. This truth becomes undeniable as group members begin recognizing how trauma lives not just in their thoughts and memories but in their muscles, breathing patterns, and nervous system responses. Sessions seven through nine shift focus from cognitive understanding to embodied awareness, helping members develop new relationships with their physical selves while building regulation skills that support all future therapeutic work.

You're moving into territory that many trauma survivors find both foreign and frightening. Years of disconnection from their bodies—often necessary for survival—have left many group members uncertain about what they feel physically or how to work with bodily sensations safely. Yet this somatic dimension holds keys to healing that purely cognitive approaches cannot access.

Body Awareness and Interoception Exercises

Interoception—the ability to sense internal bodily signals—often becomes impaired in trauma survivors who learned to disconnect from their bodies to avoid overwhelming sensations. Rebuilding this capacity requires gentle, gradual practices that help members reconnect with their physical selves without becoming overwhelmed by what they discover.

Basic body scanning provides structured entry points for developing interoceptive awareness. These exercises involve systematically attending to different body regions, noticing sensations without trying to change them, and developing vocabulary for describing physical experiences. Start with brief scans focusing on easily accessible sensations like feet contacting the floor or hands resting on legs.

Breath awareness practices help members notice their natural breathing patterns without immediately trying to change them. Many trauma survivors have developed shallow, restricted breathing patterns that limit their access to calming nervous system responses. Simply observing breath provides information about current regulation states while offering gentle entry points for developing breathing skills.

Sensation tracking involves noticing how different emotional states create physical sensations throughout the body. Members learn to recognize anger as heat or tension, anxiety as butterflies or tightness, sadness as heaviness or emptiness. This awareness helps bridge the gap between emotional and physical experiences while providing early warning systems for emotional activation.

Movement and posture awareness helps members notice how they hold themselves in space and how different postures affect their internal states. Trauma survivors often develop protective postures— shoulders raised, arms crossed, bodies positioned for escape—that reinforce hypervigilant nervous system states even in safe environments.

Comfort and discomfort differentiation teaches members to distinguish between sensations that signal safety versus danger, helping them develop trust in their bodies' wisdom while recognizing when physical sensations reflect past rather than present threats.

During Maria's first body awareness exercise, she discovered that she had been holding her breath throughout most of the group session. As she began paying attention to her breathing, she noticed shallow, restricted patterns that left her feeling anxious and lightheaded. The facilitator guided her through gentle breath awareness, helping her recognize how her body was still protecting against threats that no longer existed.

Maria also noticed chronic tension in her shoulders and jaw that she had never consciously recognized. As she began attending to these sensations, she realized they intensified during emotionally charged group discussions, providing her with valuable information about her activation levels and cues for when she might need additional grounding support.

96

The group practice of body scanning revealed diverse presentations of trauma's somatic impact. While Maria held tension in her upper body, Robert carried chronic lower back pain and digestive issues. Jennifer experienced numbness and disconnection from her body, while Michael noticed hypervigilance expressed through constant muscle readiness for action.

Gradual exposure principles ensure that body awareness practices don't overwhelm members who may have spent years avoiding bodily sensations. Start with brief exercises, focus on neutral or pleasant sensations initially, and always provide options for backing away from intense sensations without judgment.

Safety and choice become paramount in somatic work, as trauma survivors' bodies often carry memories of powerlessness and violation. All exercises should be offered as invitations rather than requirements, with clear permission to modify or stop any practice that feels unsafe or overwhelming.

Breathing Techniques and Nervous System Regulation

Breathing provides the most accessible tool for influencing nervous system states, offering immediate regulation possibilities while building long-term capacity for self-soothing. However, breathing exercises must be introduced carefully to trauma survivors, as some techniques can initially trigger anxiety or panic responses in individuals whose nervous systems are hypersensitive to internal sensations.

Natural breath observation provides the foundation for all breathing work, helping members become familiar with their current patterns before attempting any changes. This practice reduces performance anxiety while providing baseline information about individual breathing styles and restrictions.

Breath counting offers structured approaches to breathing modification that provide something concrete to focus on while developing regulation skills. Simple techniques like counting to four on the inhale and six on the exhale can activate parasympathetic nervous system responses while giving anxious minds something specific to do.

Coherent breathing involves slowing the breath to approximately five breaths per minute, creating physiological coherence between heart rate, blood pressure, and brainwave patterns. This technique, based on research by the HeartMath Institute (16), provides powerful regulation benefits while being simple enough for daily practice.

Box breathing creates equal-length inhales, holds, exhales, and holds, often in four-count patterns that provide structure and predictability. This technique, used by military and first responder training programs, helps members develop confidence in their ability to regulate their nervous systems during stressful situations.

Belly breathing helps shift from shallow chest breathing to deeper diaphragmatic breathing that activates parasympathetic responses. However, this technique must be introduced carefully, as some trauma survivors feel vulnerable or triggered by expanding their bellies, especially those with histories of sexual trauma.

Breathing modifications accommodate individual differences and trauma histories. Some members may need to breathe with eyes open, others might prefer standing rather than sitting, and those with respiratory trauma might need very gentle approaches that honor their specific sensitivities.

Robert initially resisted breathing exercises, associating them with "new age nonsense" that wouldn't help someone with "real problems." However, when the facilitator explained breathing techniques as tools used by Navy SEALs and combat medics, Robert became more willing to experiment. He discovered that box breathing helped him manage anger responses, providing him with concrete skills for staying regulated during conflicts with his wife.

The group practiced coherent breathing together, creating a shared rhythm that many members found more comforting than individual practice. This collective breathing created co-regulation experiences while reducing self-consciousness about breathing "correctly." Members reported feeling more connected to each other and more settled in their bodies after these shared practices.

Jennifer found breathing exercises initially triggered panic responses, as focusing on her breath reminded her of being unable to breathe during childhood abuse episodes. The facilitator helped her modify the practices by breathing with eyes open, focusing on external visual anchors while maintaining gentle breath awareness, and using shorter practice periods that felt manageable.

Progressive Muscle Relaxation and Grounding

Progressive muscle relaxation (PMR) provides systematic approaches to releasing chronic tension while developing awareness of the difference between tension and relaxation states. For trauma survivors who carry chronic hypervigilance in their bodies, PMR offers concrete tools for achieving physical calm while building confidence in their ability to influence their physiological states.

Traditional PMR sequences involve systematically tensing and releasing different muscle groups, starting with hands and arms and progressing through the entire body. This approach helps members recognize tension they may not have consciously noticed while teaching them how to actively create relaxation responses.

Trauma-informed modifications adapt PMR for individuals who may feel triggered by deliberately creating tension in their bodies or who may find full-body relaxation threatening. Modified approaches might focus only on releasing existing tension, work with smaller muscle groups, or maintain some alertness rather than complete relaxation.

Progressive muscle awareness involves scanning muscle groups for existing tension and gently encouraging release without first creating additional tension. This approach works well for members who find deliberate tensing triggering while still providing systematic approaches to physical relaxation.

Grounding techniques help members feel connected to the present moment and their physical environment, counteracting dissociation and anxiety responses. These techniques work with multiple sensory systems to create present-moment awareness while providing concrete anchors for consciousness.

5-4-3-2-1 grounding engages all five senses by identifying five things you can see, four things you can touch, three things you can hear, two things you can smell, and one thing you can taste. This technique provides immediate grounding while being simple enough to use in any environment.

Physical grounding uses direct contact with solid surfaces, pressure, or weight to help members feel more present in their bodies. This might include feeling feet firmly planted on the floor, pressing hands against walls or chairs, or using weighted blankets or objects during group sessions.

Environmental grounding helps members connect with their immediate surroundings through detailed observation and interaction. This approach works particularly well for members who dissociate, providing concrete tasks that require present-moment awareness while reducing overwhelming internal focus.

Lisa discovered that traditional PMR initially increased her anxiety, as deliberately tensing her muscles reminded her of bracing against physical abuse. The facilitator helped her modify the practice to focus only on releasing existing tension, using gentle movements and stretches rather than deliberate tensing and releasing.

She found particular benefit in foot grounding exercises, pressing her feet firmly into the floor while imagining roots growing from her feet into the earth. This imagery helped her feel more stable and present during emotionally intense group discussions while providing a discrete tool she could use without others noticing.

The group experimented with various grounding objects—stress balls, textured fabrics, essential oils, and small stones—discovering individual preferences for different sensory inputs. Some members preferred tactile grounding through touch, others found visual grounding through focusing on specific objects helpful, and several discovered that gentle movement provided the most effective grounding for their nervous systems.

Movement and Somatic Experiencing Adaptations

Movement provides powerful tools for processing trauma that remains stored in the body, but it must be introduced carefully to avoid overwhelming members or triggering trauma responses. Gentle, voluntary movement practices help members reconnect with their bodies while building resources for trauma processing.

Gentle stretching and mobility help members reconnect with their bodies through simple movements that release tension while building body awareness. These practices should be offered as options rather than requirements, with clear permission to modify movements based on individual comfort and safety needs.

Rhythmic movement uses repetitive, bilateral movements that can help regulate nervous system states while processing traumatic activation. Simple movements like swaying, gentle bouncing, or alternating heel lifts can provide regulation benefits while being accessible to members with different physical abilities.

Expressive movement allows members to give physical expression to emotions or internal states that may be difficult to verbalize. This might include movements that express anger, sadness, fear, or joy, helping members develop more complete emotional expression while building comfort with their bodies.

Containment and expansion exercises help members practice moving between states of protection and openness, building flexibility in their nervous system responses. These might include gentle movements that create physical boundaries followed by movements that create openness and receptivity.

Incomplete movements based on somatic experiencing principles (17) help members complete defensive responses that may have been interrupted during traumatic experiences. These practices should only be attempted with appropriate training and support, as they can access intense traumatic activation.

Dance and creative movement provide opportunities for joyful, expressive physical engagement that can help members reclaim positive relationships with their bodies. These practices should be completely voluntary and adapted to group comfort levels and individual physical abilities.

Michael initially felt self-conscious about movement exercises, associating physical expression with vulnerability that felt dangerous. However, he found that simple bilateral movements—alternating tapping his knees or gentle swaying—helped him stay present during emotionally difficult group discussions while providing outlets for activation energy.

The group experimented with standing and gentle movement during check-ins, discovering that many members felt more comfortable sharing while moving slightly rather than sitting still. This discovery led to incorporating optional movement into various group activities, honoring different members' needs for physical expression and regulation.

Sarah found that gentle stretching helped her access emotions that felt stuck in her body, particularly anger that she had learned to suppress during childhood. Through careful exploration with group support, she began using movement to help express and release emotions that had been trapped in chronic muscle tension.

Window of Tolerance Expansion Practices

The window of tolerance—the zone where individuals can experience emotions and sensations without becoming overwhelmed or shutting down—provides a central framework for all somatic work. Expanding this window requires gradual, supported experiences of intensity that build resilience without overwhelming the nervous system.

Tolerance building exercises involve deliberately practicing with manageable levels of activation while maintaining present-moment awareness and regulation skills. These exercises help members build confidence in their ability to handle increasing levels of intensity without becoming dysregulated.

Edge work involves carefully approaching the boundaries of comfort zones while maintaining support and safety. Members learn to recognize their edges—points where they begin feeling overwhelmed—while practicing staying present at these thresholds rather than immediately backing away.

Pendulation practices help members move between activated and settled states, building flexibility in their nervous system responses while developing skills for self-regulation. These practices teach members that activation states are temporary and that they can influence their physiological responses.

Resource building involves identifying and practicing access to internal and external resources that support regulation and resilience. Resources might include supportive relationships, calming environments, positive memories, spiritual practices, or specific activities that promote wellbeing.

Titrated exposure provides graduated approaches to working with difficult sensations or emotions, starting with very small doses and gradually increasing intensity as tolerance builds. This approach respects the nervous system's capacity while promoting growth and healing.

Integration practices help members consolidate learning from somatic experiences while building meaning and understanding around their physical responses. This integration bridges somatic and cognitive approaches to healing while helping members apply insights to daily life.

David discovered through window of tolerance work that his range of comfortable experience was extremely narrow—he felt anxious when experiencing any strong emotion, whether positive or negative. Through gradual practice with group support, he began expanding his capacity to tolerate joy, anger, sadness, and excitement without immediately shutting down or becoming overwhelmed.

The group practiced together with pendulation exercises, learning to move between states of activation and calm while supporting each other through the experience. These shared practices created safety while helping members build tolerance for intensity that previously felt overwhelming.

Jennifer worked specifically with expanding her tolerance for pleasant sensations, as trauma had taught her to be suspicious of positive experiences that might be followed by pain or violation. Through careful practice, she began allowing herself to fully experience moments of connection, laughter, and physical comfort without immediately bracing for danger.

Building Somatic Resources for Trauma Processing

The somatic awareness and regulation skills developed during these sessions provide essential foundations for the trauma processing work that follows. Members need solid grounding in body awareness and self-regulation before they can safely approach traumatic memories and their associated physiological responses.

Regulation skill mastery ensures that members have reliable tools for managing activation before they begin processing traumatic material. These skills include breathing techniques, grounding practices, movement resources, and awareness of their window of tolerance boundaries.

Body literacy development helps members understand and trust their physical responses while developing language for describing somatic experiences. This literacy becomes essential for trauma processing, as much of traumatic experience is stored in pre-verbal, somatic form.

Co-regulation experiences within the group help members practice using interpersonal connection for nervous system regulation, building skills they'll need for healing traumatic material that often involves relational wounding.

Safety signal development helps members recognize and create environmental and interpersonal cues that signal safety to their nervous systems, providing resources for managing triggering situations both in and outside of group sessions.

Resilience building involves identifying and strengthening factors that support members' capacity to handle challenging experiences while recovering from difficulties. These might include physical practices, social connections, spiritual resources, or creative activities that promote wellbeing.

The transformation in group members' relationship with their bodies often becomes evident during these sessions. Members who arrived feeling disconnected from or fearful of their physical selves begin developing curiosity about their somatic experiences. Those who carried chronic tension begin experiencing moments of relaxation and ease.

Most importantly, members begin trusting their bodies as sources of information and resources rather than just sources of symptoms and problems. This shift in relationship provides the foundation for trauma processing, as members develop confidence in their ability to navigate difficult material while maintaining connection to their resources and support.

Embodied Healing

The somatic work of sessions seven through nine represents more than skill-building—it's a reclamation process. Trauma survivors are reconnecting with aspects of themselves that were lost or buried in the aftermath of overwhelming experiences. They're learning to inhabit their bodies fully while honoring both their vulnerabilities and their strengths.

This embodied approach to healing recognizes that trauma impacts the whole person—mind, body, and spirit—and that lasting recovery requires addressing all these dimensions. The nervous system regulation skills developed during these sessions will support every aspect of future group work while providing tools for lifelong wellbeing.

The group often becomes more cohesive during these sessions as members share vulnerable experiences of reconnecting with their bodies. Witnessing each other's courage in facing physical sensations that have been avoided for years creates deep bonds while providing models of gentle self-compassion and acceptance.

Key Learning Outcomes

- Body awareness and interoception exercises help trauma survivors reconnect with physical sensations safely and gradually
- Breathing techniques provide immediate regulation tools while building long-term nervous system flexibility and resilience
- Progressive muscle relaxation and grounding practices offer concrete methods for releasing chronic tension and staying present
- Movement and somatic experiencing adaptations help members process trauma stored in the body through gentle physical expression
- Window of tolerance expansion practices build capacity for experiencing intensity without becoming overwhelmed or shutting down
- These somatic foundations become essential resources for trauma processing while supporting overall regulation and wellbeing
-

Chapter 10: Processing Traumatic Memories Through Imagery (Sessions 10-12)

Memory lives in layers—conscious narratives that we can speak about, wordless sensations that grip our bodies, and images that flash through awareness carrying the full emotional weight of past experiences. Sessions ten through twelve bring group members face-to-face with these memory layers, using carefully structured imagery work to process traumatic experiences in ways that promote healing rather than retraumatization.

This phase of group work requires everything you've built in previous sessions—safety, regulation skills, group cohesion, and somatic awareness. Without these foundations, imagery work can become overwhelming or dangerous. With them, it becomes one of the most powerful tools available for transforming traumatic experiences from sources of ongoing distress into integrated aspects of personal history.

Safety Protocols for Trauma Processing

Processing traumatic memories in group settings requires robust safety protocols that protect both individual members and group integrity. These protocols must address the reality that trauma processing can trigger intense reactions while maintaining the support and witnessing that make group work uniquely healing.

Pre-processing assessment determines individual readiness for trauma-focused work by evaluating current stability, regulation skills, support systems, and motivation for processing. Not all group members will be ready for intensive trauma work at the same time, and individualized timing prevents overwhelm while honoring different healing paces.

Informed consent ensures that members understand what trauma processing involves, potential risks and benefits, their right to control the process, and available support resources. This consent should be ongoing rather than one-time, as members' comfort levels may change as work progresses.

Dosing and titration involve working with manageable pieces of traumatic experience rather than attempting to process entire traumatic events at once. This approach respects the nervous system's capacity for integration while preventing flooding that can retraumatize rather than heal.

Dual awareness maintenance helps members stay connected to both past experiences and present safety while processing traumatic memories. This skill prevents complete immersion in traumatic states while allowing sufficient engagement for healing to occur.

Grounding and regulation resources must be immediately available during trauma processing, including co-regulation from facilitators and group members, environmental anchors, and personal regulation tools that members have practiced extensively.

Processing limits establish clear boundaries around how much traumatic material will be processed in single sessions, ensuring that members don't become overwhelmed while maintaining sufficient time for integration and stabilization before sessions end.

When Jennifer prepared to process childhood sexual abuse memories, the facilitator spent considerable time establishing safety protocols specific to her needs. Jennifer needed to sit where she could see the door, preferred to keep her eyes partially open during imagery work, and wanted permission to stop the process at any time without explanation or pressure to continue.

The group developed specific agreements about how to support Jennifer during her processing work—maintaining quiet, attentive presence without trying to rescue or fix her experience, offering gentle grounding reminders if she appeared to dissociate, and providing validation and witnessing after she completed her work.

These protocols were tested during Jennifer's first imagery session when she became overwhelmed and began hyperventilating. The facilitator immediately helped her return to present-moment awareness through grounding techniques while group members provided calm, supportive presence. This experience reinforced the importance of safety protocols while demonstrating the group's capacity to contain difficult material.

Imagery Rescripting in Group Format

Imagery rescripting allows group members to revisit traumatic experiences with adult resources, changing helpless victim narratives into stories of survival, strength, and recovery. This technique must be adapted for group settings in ways that maximize therapeutic benefits while maintaining safety for all participants.

Memory selection involves choosing specific traumatic experiences that are appropriate for group processing. Generally, this means avoiding memories that are too overwhelming, too private, or likely to trigger other group members excessively. The focus should be on memories that represent themes or patterns rather than the most extreme traumatic events.

Scene setting helps members establish the traumatic memory scenario in sufficient detail to access the emotional material while maintaining enough distance to stay regulated. This process requires careful balance between engagement and overwhelm, often starting with peripheral details before approaching core elements.

Resource identification involves helping members recognize internal and external resources they can bring to the traumatic scenario. These might include current adult knowledge and skills, supportive relationships, spiritual resources, or simply the knowledge that they survived the experience and are now safe.

Rescripting process allows members to reimagine the traumatic scenario with their adult resources available, changing outcomes, providing protection to their younger selves, or simply offering comfort and validation to the part of them that endured the trauma.

Integration and meaning-making help members understand how the rescripting experience changes their relationship to the traumatic memory while identifying insights or resources that can be applied to current life situations.

Group witnessing provides the collective holding and validation that makes group rescripting particularly powerful. Members experience having their traumatic experiences witnessed and honored by others while receiving support for their strength and resilience in surviving difficult circumstances.

Robert chose to process a combat memory involving the death of a fellow soldier in an IED explosion. Rather than processing the most traumatic aspects of the event, he focused on his feelings of helplessness and responsibility for his friend's death. The rescripting work involved imagining himself providing comfort to his dying friend while receiving support from other soldiers.

During the rescripting, Robert was able to tell his friend that his death wasn't Robert's fault, that he was loved and valued, and that Robert would carry his memory with honor. The group witnessed Robert's grief and love for his fallen comrade while supporting his movement from self-blame toward acceptance and meaning-making.

This processing experience helped Robert understand that survivor guilt was a normal response to combat loss while reducing the intensity of shame and self-blame he'd carried for years. The group's witnessing of his love and grief helped validate his loss while honoring his friend's memory.

Witness Consciousness and Group Support

The power of group imagery work lies partly in the collective witnessing that occurs as members share their traumatic experiences with others who understand trauma's impact. This witnessing must be structured carefully to provide healing support while avoiding overwhelm or secondary traumatization of group members.

Witness preparation helps group members understand their role as compassionate observers who provide presence and support without trying to fix or change others' experiences. This preparation includes managing their own emotional responses while maintaining supportive presence for processing members.

Supportive presence involves maintaining calm, attentive awareness while members process traumatic material. This presence should be non-judgmental, non-intrusive, and focused on providing safe holding for whatever emerges during processing work.

Co-regulation provision occurs naturally as regulated group members help support the nervous systems of members who are processing traumatic material. This co-regulation happens through presence, breathing, and energetic attunement rather than through direct intervention.

Validation and normalization help processing members understand that their traumatic experiences and responses make sense while reducing shame and isolation. This validation should acknowledge both the reality of traumatic events and the strength required to survive them.

Boundary maintenance ensures that witness group members don't become overwhelmed by others' traumatic material while maintaining appropriate emotional boundaries. Members learn to provide support while taking care of their own emotional needs and regulation.

Post-processing support involves offering appropriate acknowledgment and appreciation for members' courage in sharing traumatic experiences while helping them integrate insights from their processing work.

During Maria's processing of childhood abuse memories, the group provided powerful witnessing that helped transform her experience of shame and isolation. As she worked through memories of being blamed and silenced by family members, group members offered validation that she was not responsible for the abuse and that her survival represented incredible strength.

The group's collective presence helped Maria feel that her experience mattered and that she deserved support and care. This witnessing experience challenged her core beliefs about being worthless and undeserving while providing corrective experiences of being seen and valued by others.

Several group members shared that witnessing Maria's courage in processing her trauma helped them recognize their own strength and resilience. This mutual benefit illustrates how group processing creates healing opportunities for both processing and witnessing members.

Managing Dissociation and Overwhelm

Trauma processing naturally activates defensive responses, including dissociation and overwhelm, that protected individuals during original traumatic experiences. Managing these responses requires sophisticated understanding of trauma's impact on consciousness while maintaining safety and therapeutic progress.

Dissociation recognition involves identifying when group members disconnect from present-moment awareness during trauma processing. Signs might include blank stares, unresponsiveness to verbal contact, dramatic changes in vocal tone or body posture, or reports of feeling "spacey" or "not here."

Grounding interventions help dissociated members return to present-moment awareness through sensory anchoring, bilateral stimulation, movement, or verbal orientation. These interventions should be gentle and non-demanding while providing clear pathways back to current reality.

Overwhelm management addresses situations where members become flooded with emotional or physiological activation that exceeds their window of tolerance. Management strategies include slowing down the process, increasing grounding and support, or temporarily stopping trauma processing to focus on regulation.

Pacing and titration prevent dissociation and overwhelm by working with small pieces of traumatic experience while maintaining connection to present-moment resources. This approach respects the nervous system's capacity for integration while promoting healing rather than retraumatization.

Support escalation provides graduated levels of intervention based on members' needs, starting with gentle redirection and potentially escalating to more intensive grounding or crisis intervention if necessary.

Recovery and integration help members return to regulated states after managing dissociation or overwhelm while integrating any insights or progress that occurred during the processing work.

David experienced significant dissociation during his first trauma processing session, appearing to "leave" his body completely while accessing memories of childhood emotional abuse. The facilitator noticed his blank stare and unresponsiveness to verbal contact, immediately implementing grounding interventions.

Using his name repeatedly, asking him to feel his feet on the floor, and providing bilateral stimulation through gentle tapping, the facilitator helped David return to present-moment awareness. The group provided supportive presence while David reoriented to current reality, expressing appreciation for his courage while acknowledging the difficulty of trauma processing.

This experience taught David to recognize early signs of dissociation while developing strategies for staying more present during trauma processing. Subsequent sessions involved more careful pacing and increased grounding support, allowing him to process traumatic material without losing connection to current safety.

Integration and Meaning-Making Processes

The therapeutic value of trauma processing lies not just in emotional expression but in the integration and meaning-making that transform traumatic experiences from sources of ongoing distress into integrated aspects of personal history. This integration requires time, support, and structured processes that help members make sense of their experiences.

Immediate integration occurs directly after trauma processing through gentle discussion of what occurred, validation of members' courage and strength, and initial exploration of insights or changes that resulted from the processing work.

Somatic integration helps members notice how trauma processing affected their bodies, potentially releasing chronic tension, changing breathing patterns, or creating new sensations of groundedness or openness. These physical changes often indicate successful trauma processing at nervous system levels.

Cognitive integration involves helping members understand how trauma processing changes their thoughts, beliefs, or perspectives about themselves, others, or their traumatic experiences. This integration bridges emotional processing with cognitive understanding while promoting lasting change.

Narrative integration helps members develop coherent stories about their traumatic experiences that acknowledge both the reality of what happened and their strength in surviving and healing. These narratives should honor the truth of traumatic experiences while emphasizing resilience and recovery.

Relational integration explores how trauma processing affects members' relationships with others, potentially increasing capacity for intimacy, trust, or emotional expression. Group processing often directly impacts relational patterns as members practice vulnerability and receive support.

Spiritual integration may involve exploring how traumatic experiences and healing processes affect members' sense of meaning, purpose, or connection to something larger than themselves. This integration should respect diverse spiritual perspectives while honoring the spiritual dimensions of healing.

Lisa's processing of childhood neglect memories led to significant integration work around her patterns of caretaking and self-neglect. Through imagery rescripting, she was able to provide the comfort and attention to her younger self that had been missing from her actual childhood experience.

This processing work helped Lisa recognize that her adult caretaking patterns represented attempts to give others what she had needed as a child. While this pattern had positive aspects, it also led to exhaustion and resentment when her own needs remained unmet. The integration work helped her develop more balanced approaches to caring for both herself and others.

The group supported Lisa's integration by providing feedback about changes they observed in her self-advocacy and boundary-setting. This relational feedback helped reinforce the insights from her trauma processing while providing ongoing support for implementing changes in her daily life.

Building Resilience Through Processing

Trauma processing, when conducted safely and skillfully, builds resilience rather than retraumatization. Group members discover their capacity to face difficult material while maintaining connection to current resources and support. This discovery transforms their relationship to their traumatic experiences while building confidence in their ability to handle life's challenges.

Post-traumatic growth often emerges through trauma processing as members discover strengths, resources, and capacities they didn't know they possessed. This growth doesn't minimize traumatic experiences but demonstrates the human capacity for healing and transformation in the face of adversity.

Resource development continues as members identify internal and external resources that supported them during traumatic experiences and continue to support their healing. These resources become available for managing current challenges while building resilience for future difficulties.

Mastery experiences occur as members successfully process traumatic material without becoming overwhelmed or retraumatized. These experiences build confidence in their healing capacity while reducing fear of their own emotional responses and memories.

Narrative coherence develops as traumatic experiences become integrated into coherent life stories that include both suffering and healing, victimization and survival, wounding and growth. These coherent narratives support psychological health while honoring the complexity of human experience.

Meaning-making helps members find purpose and significance in their traumatic experiences and healing journeys. This meaning-making doesn't justify trauma but helps members understand how their experiences can contribute to their own growth and their ability to help others.

The group process itself becomes a source of resilience as members witness each other's courage in facing traumatic material while providing mutual support through difficult healing work. These shared experiences create bonds that often extend beyond formal group treatment while providing models of healthy relationships and support.

Honoring the Journey

Trauma processing represents sacred work—the transformation of pain into wisdom, victimization into empowerment, isolation into connection. Group members who engage in this work demonstrate remarkable courage while supporting each other through some of life's most difficult territory.

The imagery work of sessions ten through twelve often marks a turning point in group treatment as members begin experiencing themselves as survivors rather than victims, as resilient individuals rather than damaged goods. This shift in identity provides foundations for all future healing work while opening possibilities for post-traumatic growth.

The witnessing and support that occurs during group trauma processing creates healing opportunities that individual therapy cannot replicate. Members experience having their most difficult experiences validated and honored by others while discovering their own capacity to support others through similar struggles.

Important Takeaways

- Robust safety protocols ensure trauma processing promotes healing rather than retraumatization while protecting all group members
- Imagery rescripting allows members to revisit traumatic experiences with adult resources while changing victim narratives into survival stories
- Group witnessing provides powerful validation and support that transforms shame and isolation into connection and understanding
- Managing dissociation and overwhelm requires sophisticated interventions that maintain safety while supporting therapeutic progress
- Integration and meaning-making processes transform traumatic experiences from sources of distress into integrated aspects of personal history
- Trauma processing builds resilience and post-traumatic growth while demonstrating members' capacity for healing and transformation

Chapter 11: Chair Work and Parts Integration (Sessions 13-15)

The empty chair sits in the center of the group circle like a portal between worlds—a space where past and present converge, where wounded parts of the self can finally speak their truth, and where healing conversations that never happened in real life can unfold with profound therapeutic power. Sessions thirteen through fifteen introduce group members to chair work and parts integration, techniques that help them access, dialogue with, and heal the different aspects of themselves that were fragmented by traumatic experiences.

This work requires tremendous courage. Group members must be willing to speak to and for parts of themselves that may have been buried for decades, to give voice to pain that has been silenced, and to engage in conversations with internal figures who may have caused great harm. Yet this courage is rewarded with integration, self-compassion, and the profound relief that comes from no longer fighting internal wars.

Empty Chair Techniques for Trauma Work

Chair work provides concrete, experiential approaches to trauma processing that access emotional and somatic material often unavailable through traditional talk therapy. The empty chair becomes a safe space for encounters with traumatic memories, internal conflicts, and relationship dynamics that continue affecting current life experiences.

Basic chair work setup involves placing an empty chair in the group space where members can imagine significant others, younger versions of themselves, or internal parts sitting. This physical representation makes internal experiences more concrete while providing clear focus for therapeutic work.

Safety and preparation ensure that chair work doesn't overwhelm members or trigger uncontrolled emotional responses. Preparation includes establishing grounding resources, clarifying session goals, and ensuring adequate time for integration after intensive emotional work.

Dialogue facilitation helps members engage in genuine conversations with whoever they place in the empty chair, encouraging authentic expression while maintaining therapeutic safety. The facilitator serves as guide and witness while avoiding excessive direction that might interfere with members' natural processes.

Role switching allows members to speak both as themselves and as whoever they've placed in the chair, providing opportunities to explore different perspectives while accessing empathy and understanding for various viewpoints.

Processing and integration help members understand insights gained through chair work while connecting these experiences to current life patterns and relationships. This integration bridges experimental work with practical application in daily life.

Group witnessing provides collective support and validation for chair work while offering feedback about changes group members observe during these intensive experiences.

Sarah chose to use chair work to process her relationship with her deceased mother, whose critical voice continued affecting her self-esteem years after her mother's death. Sarah placed her mother in the empty chair and began expressing feelings she'd never been able to share while her mother was alive.

"You never told me you loved me," Sarah said to the empty chair, her voice shaking with decades of suppressed pain. "I spent my whole childhood trying to make you proud, but nothing I did was ever good enough. I needed you to see me, to value me, to tell me I mattered."

When the facilitator encouraged Sarah to switch chairs and respond as her mother, she initially resisted, feeling disloyal to her own pain. However, speaking from her mother's perspective helped Sarah recognize that her mother's criticism reflected her own insecurities and fears rather than Sarah's inadequacies.

This chair work helped Sarah begin separating her mother's issues from her own worth while developing compassion for both her mother's struggles and her own childhood pain. The group's witnessing of this process provided validation for Sarah's experience while supporting her growing self-compassion.

Internal Family Systems Adaptations

Internal Family Systems (IFS) theory, developed by Richard Schwartz (18), provides frameworks for understanding the different parts of personality that develop in response to life experiences, particularly traumatic ones. Adapting IFS concepts for group settings creates opportunities for parts work while leveraging group support and witnessing.

Parts identification helps members recognize the different aspects of their personalities that emerged to handle various life circumstances. These parts often include protectors (who try to prevent future hurt), exiles (who carry painful emotions and memories), and firefighters (who try to distract from or numb overwhelming experiences).

Self-energy cultivation involves accessing the core self that exists beneath protective parts—the aspect of personality that is naturally curious, compassionate, courageous, and calm. This self-energy provides the internal resource necessary for healing wounded parts while maintaining healthy boundaries.

Parts mapping creates visual or descriptive representations of members' internal systems, helping them understand how different parts interact and influence their daily experiences. This mapping process often reveals parts that have been hidden or disowned due to shame or fear.

Parts appreciation involves recognizing the positive intentions behind even problematic parts, understanding that protective

120

mechanisms developed for important reasons even when they now create difficulties. This appreciation reduces internal conflict while opening possibilities for negotiating new arrangements between parts.

Unburdening work helps wounded parts release pain and trauma they've been carrying, often for decades. This process requires patience, compassion, and skilled facilitation to ensure that parts feel ready and safe to let go of their protective roles.

Integration practices help members coordinate their various parts in service of healthy adult functioning, with self-energy leading the internal system while honoring the contributions and concerns of different parts.

Michael discovered through parts work that he had a young protector part that became hypervigilant during childhood to keep him safe from his unpredictable, alcoholic father. This part constantly scanned for danger, interrupted his sleep with worry, and made it difficult for him to relax even in safe environments.

He also identified an exile part that carried the terror and helplessness from childhood abuse experiences. This part had been locked away to prevent overwhelming pain but continued affecting his ability to be vulnerable in relationships. Additionally, he recognized a firefighter part that used work addiction to distract from emotional pain.

Through group parts work, Michael began developing relationships with these different aspects of himself, appreciating their protective intentions while helping them recognize that he was now safe and had adult resources for handling difficulties. This internal negotiation reduced his chronic anxiety while improving his capacity for intimate relationships.

Dialoguing with Protective and Wounded Parts

Parts dialogue provides structured approaches for communicating with different aspects of the self, healing internal conflicts, and developing more harmonious internal relationships. This work often reveals that internal criticism and conflict reflect attempts at protection rather than genuine self-hatred.

Protective parts dialogue involves communicating with parts that developed to prevent future hurt or harm. These parts often carry heavy burdens of responsibility and may resist change due to fears about safety and survival. Dialogue helps these parts feel heard while exploring possibilities for updating their roles.

Wounded parts dialogue provides opportunities for exiled parts to express pain that may have been suppressed for years or decades. These conversations require patience and compassion, as wounded parts may initially be reluctant to trust that it's safe to share their experiences.

Mediating internal conflicts helps resolve battles between different parts that may have opposing goals or strategies. These conflicts often reflect normal responses to complex circumstances where different survival strategies were needed simultaneously.

Reparenting wounded parts allows members' adult selves to provide comfort, protection, and validation that wounded parts needed but didn't receive during traumatic experiences. This reparenting process helps heal developmental wounds while building internal resources for self-care and resilience.

Setting internal boundaries involves negotiating agreements between parts about roles, responsibilities, and appropriate times for different parts to be active. These boundaries help prevent parts from overwhelming each other while ensuring that all parts' needs are considered.

Developing internal cooperation creates collaborative relationships between parts rather than competitive or conflictual ones. This cooperation allows members to access the strengths of different parts while maintaining overall internal harmony and effective functioning.

Jennifer's parts dialogue revealed intense conflict between a perfectionist part that demanded flawless performance and a rebellious part that wanted to reject all expectations and standards. These parts had been battling for years, leaving Jennifer exhausted and feeling torn between extremes.

Through guided dialogue, Jennifer helped these parts understand each other's concerns. The perfectionist part feared that any mistakes would lead to abandonment or criticism, drawing from childhood experiences of conditional love. The rebellious part was exhausted from impossible standards and wanted freedom to be human and imperfect.

The group witnessed Jennifer's internal negotiation as she helped these parts develop a cooperative agreement. The perfectionist part agreed to set realistic standards while the rebellious part committed to making thoughtful choices rather than reactive rejections of all expectations. This internal peace translated into reduced anxiety and more balanced approaches to work and relationships.

Group Witnessing of Parts Work

The collective witnessing that occurs during group parts work provides validation and normalization for internal experiences that members may have kept private due to shame or fear of being misunderstood. This witnessing helps reduce isolation while providing models for healthy internal relationships.

Witnessing guidelines help group members provide supportive presence during parts work without interfering with individuals' natural processes. This includes maintaining respectful attention, avoiding advice-giving or interpretation, and offering appreciation for members' courage in exploring internal dynamics.

Normalization benefits occur as group members recognize similar parts and internal conflicts in each other's presentations. This recognition reduces shame about internal complexity while demonstrating that parts development represents normal responses to life circumstances.

Modeling opportunities emerge as group members observe different approaches to parts dialogue and internal negotiation. These observations provide ideas and inspiration for members' own parts work while demonstrating various pathways to internal healing.

Feedback and reflection help members understand how their parts work affects others, providing valuable information about interpersonal patterns while building awareness of their impact on relationships.

Collective healing occurs as group members' parts work affects the entire group system, often activating similar parts in other members while providing opportunities for mutual support and understanding.

Integration support helps members process insights from parts work while developing plans for applying new internal arrangements to daily life situations.

When Robert engaged in parts work around his combat trauma, he identified a warrior part that had served him well during military service but created problems in civilian relationships. This part was hypervigilant, aggressive, and suspicious of others' motives—qualities that kept him alive in combat but interfered with intimacy and trust.

The group witnessed Robert's appreciation for this warrior part's service while helping it understand that civilian life required different strategies. Other group members shared their own experiences with parts that served important functions in traumatic situations but needed updating for current circumstances.

This collective witnessing helped normalize Robert's experience while providing support for his internal negotiation process. The group's understanding and acceptance helped reduce his shame about aggressive impulses while supporting his development of more flexible responses to perceived threats.

Integration Exercises and Homework Assignments

Parts integration requires ongoing practice between sessions as members learn to recognize parts activation in daily life while implementing new internal arrangements. Integration exercises provide structured approaches for maintaining parts work progress while building skills for independent parts management.

Parts check-ins involve brief daily practices of noticing which parts are active and what they might need. These check-ins help members maintain awareness of internal dynamics while preventing parts from becoming overwhelmed or taking control unconsciously.

Internal negotiation practice helps members mediate parts conflicts as they arise in daily life, using skills developed during group sessions to resolve internal disagreements without becoming paralyzed or overwhelmed.

Self-energy cultivation involves practices that help members access and maintain connection to their core self, the aspect of personality that can provide internal leadership and coordination. These practices might include meditation, journaling, creative expression, or spiritual activities.

Parts appreciation exercises help members maintain positive relationships with all parts, even those that create difficulties. This appreciation prevents internal rejection and conflict while promoting cooperation and integration.

Boundary setting practice involves implementing agreements developed during parts work, helping members maintain internal balance while preventing parts from overwhelming each other or taking control inappropriately.

Integration journaling provides structured approaches for tracking parts work progress while processing insights and challenges that emerge during daily implementation of new internal arrangements.

Lisa developed a daily parts check-in practice where she would briefly notice which parts were active and what they might need before making important decisions. This practice helped her recognize when her people-pleasing part was taking control without input from other parts of herself.

She also practiced internal negotiation when conflicts arose between her caretaking part and her part that wanted personal time and space. Rather than automatically defaulting to caretaking, Lisa learned to facilitate internal discussions that honored both parts' concerns while finding creative solutions.

Her homework included writing letters between different parts, helping them communicate more effectively while building understanding and cooperation. This correspondence helped Lisa maintain the internal harmony developed during group sessions while building skills for independent parts management.

Advanced Parts Work Techniques

As group members develop comfort with basic parts dialogue, more sophisticated techniques become available for addressing complex internal dynamics and stubborn patterns that resist initial intervention attempts.

Parts restructuring involves helping parts take on new roles or responsibilities that better serve members' current life circumstances. This restructuring process requires patience and negotiation, as parts may resist changing roles that have provided safety and identity.

Parts unburdening ceremonies provide ritual approaches to helping parts release pain, responsibilities, or roles that no longer serve healthy functioning. These ceremonies should be conducted with appropriate reverence and support, recognizing the significance of parts' service and sacrifice.

Parts strengths integration helps members access positive qualities that different parts possess, building on parts' resources rather than focusing only on problems or conflicts. This integration creates more balanced internal systems while appreciating parts' contributions.

Trauma-specific parts work addresses parts that developed specifically in response to traumatic experiences, helping them process and integrate traumatic material while updating their protective strategies for current circumstances.

Somatic parts work incorporates body awareness and movement into parts dialogue, recognizing that parts often express themselves through physical sensations, postures, and movements. This somatic dimension adds depth and authenticity to parts work while providing additional channels for communication.

Creative parts expression uses art, music, movement, or creative writing to help parts express themselves in non-verbal ways. These creative approaches often access parts material that remains unavailable through traditional dialogue while providing enjoyable and engaging healing experiences.

David engaged in advanced parts work around a part that carried shame about his childhood sexual abuse. This part had been hidden for decades, creating depression and self-hatred while interfering with his ability to form intimate relationships.

Through careful, patient work with group support, David helped this wounded part express its pain and shame while providing the protection and validation it had never received. The group witnessed this courageous work while offering appreciation for both David's strength and the part's survival through impossible circumstances.

This unburdening work helped the wounded part release decades of carried pain while allowing David to access compassion for his childhood experience. The integration of this previously hidden part contributed to reduced depression while improving his capacity for vulnerability and connection in relationships.

Building Internal Harmony

Parts work aims not to eliminate problematic parts but to create internal harmony where all parts can contribute their strengths while cooperating with overall healthy functioning. This harmony requires ongoing attention and maintenance as life circumstances change and new challenges emerge.

Internal democracy involves ensuring that all parts have voice and representation in internal decision-making while maintaining appropriate leadership from self-energy. This democratic approach prevents parts from feeling suppressed or ignored while maintaining effective internal coordination.

Parts appreciation practices help maintain positive relationships with all aspects of the self, even those that sometimes create difficulties. This appreciation reduces internal conflict while promoting cooperation and mutual support between parts.

Flexible parts activation allows different parts to take leadership in appropriate situations while maintaining overall internal coordination. This flexibility helps members adapt to various life circumstances while preventing any single part from dominating their entire personality.

Internal conflict resolution provides ongoing skills for managing disagreements between parts as they arise, preventing internal battles from paralyzing decision-making or creating overwhelming internal tension.

Parts boundary maintenance ensures that parts respect each other's roles and territories while preventing inappropriate interference or takeover attempts. These boundaries support internal stability while allowing for appropriate parts collaboration.

Integration monitoring involves tracking how well internal systems are functioning while identifying areas that may need additional attention or adjustment. This monitoring helps prevent regression while supporting continued internal development.

The group often becomes a laboratory for practicing internal integration as members experiment with allowing different parts to be present and active during group interactions. This practice provides valuable feedback about how internal changes affect interpersonal relationships while building confidence in new internal arrangements.

Moving Toward Wholeness

Parts work represents a journey toward internal integration and wholeness that honors the complexity of human personality while healing the fragmentation that trauma creates. Group members learn to appreciate all aspects of themselves while developing internal leadership that can coordinate their various parts effectively.

This integration work often reveals that members are more complex, resourceful, and capable than they previously recognized. Parts that seemed problematic often contain valuable qualities and strengths that can contribute to healthy functioning when properly integrated and coordinated.

The group witnessing of parts work creates powerful healing experiences as members observe each other's courage in facing internal complexity while providing mutual support for integration processes. These shared experiences often deepen group bonds while providing models for healthy internal and external relationships.

The internal harmony developed through parts work provides foundations for the remaining phases of group treatment, as members become more capable of managing intense emotions, processing difficult material, and maintaining healthy relationships with themselves and others.

Essential Elements for Growth

- Empty chair techniques provide concrete, experiential approaches to processing trauma and internal conflicts through dialogue and role-switching
- Internal Family Systems adaptations help members identify, understand, and develop healthy relationships with different aspects of their personalities

- Parts dialogue facilitates communication between protective and wounded parts while mediating internal conflicts and building cooperation
- Group witnessing provides validation and normalization for parts work while offering modeling opportunities and integration support
- Integration exercises and homework assignments help members maintain parts work progress while building skills for independent internal management
- Advanced techniques address complex internal dynamics while incorporating somatic, creative, and trauma-specific approaches to parts integration

Chapter 12: Addressing Shame and the Punitive Parent Mode (Sessions 16-18)

Shame whispers its poison in the quiet moments—you're not good enough, you don't deserve love, you should be able to handle this alone. For trauma survivors, shame often becomes the central organizing principle around which their entire sense of self revolves. Sessions sixteen through eighteen tackle this most corrosive emotion directly, helping group members distinguish between healthy guilt (which motivates positive change) and toxic shame (which attacks the very core of their being).

The punitive parent mode carries shame's voice, delivering harsh criticisms and impossible standards learned from childhood experiences of conditional love, criticism, or abuse. This internal critic may sound like actual caregivers from the past, or it may represent internalized cultural messages about worthiness, success, and acceptability. Regardless of its origins, the punitive parent mode creates ongoing internal abuse that maintains trauma symptoms long after external threats have ended.

Understanding Toxic Shame vs. Healthy Guilt

The distinction between shame and guilt represents one of the most important concepts in trauma recovery, yet many survivors have never learned to differentiate between these vastly different emotional experiences. Understanding this difference provides the foundation for all shame-healing work that follows.

Healthy guilt focuses on specific behaviors or actions, creating emotional discomfort that motivates positive change while preserving self-worth. Guilt says "I did something bad" and generally leads to repair attempts, apologies, or behavior change. This emotion serves important social and moral functions by helping individuals recognize when their actions have caused harm.

Toxic shame attacks the entire self, creating global feelings of worthlessness, defectiveness, or badness that extend far beyond specific actions. Shame says "I am bad" and typically leads to hiding, withdrawal, or self-attack rather than positive change. This emotion serves no useful function and actively interferes with healing and growth.

Shame's physiological impact includes decreased immune function, elevated stress hormones, increased inflammation, and disrupted nervous system regulation. Chronic shame literally makes people sick while interfering with their ability to think clearly, form relationships, or make positive life changes.

Cultural and family shame messages often become internalized during childhood when individuals lack the developmental capacity to question or resist these messages. Children naturally assume that treatment they receive reflects their worth, leading to deep shame when they experience abuse, neglect, or criticism.

Trauma-related shame emerges when individuals blame themselves for traumatic experiences, survival strategies they used, or their ongoing symptoms and struggles. This self-blame compounds trauma's impact while interfering with healing and recovery processes.

Internalized oppression creates shame in individuals from marginalized groups who absorb negative societal messages about their identities. This systemic shame adds additional layers to trauma-related shame while requiring attention to both individual and cultural healing.

Maria's shame work revealed how deeply she had internalized messages from her childhood sexual abuse experience. She carried profound shame about "letting" the abuse happen, about not telling anyone sooner, and about the ways the trauma continued affecting her adult relationships and sexuality.

Through group discussion, Maria began recognizing that her shame reflected normal childhood responses to abnormal circumstances rather than evidence of her defectiveness or culpability. The group helped her understand that children cannot consent to sexual activity and that her survival strategies represented resourcefulness rather than complicity.

The facilitator helped Maria distinguish between appropriate sadness about what happened to her (healthy emotional response) and shame about being the kind of person to whom such things happen (toxic self-attack). This distinction helped Maria begin directing her emotional energy toward healing rather than self-punishment.

Identifying Internalized Critical Voices

The punitive parent mode often operates automatically, delivering harsh criticisms and impossible standards without conscious recognition or challenge. Learning to identify these internal voices represents the first step toward developing more compassionate internal relationships.

Voice identification exercises help group members recognize specific critical messages they deliver to themselves while distinguishing between their authentic voice and internalized others. These exercises often reveal that internal criticism sounds remarkably similar to childhood caregivers, teachers, or cultural authorities.

Content analysis examines what punitive parent voices say, revealing common themes like worthlessness, inadequacy, responsibility for others' behavior, impossible standards, or predictions of failure and rejection. Understanding these themes helps members recognize patterns while developing targeted responses.

Tone and language examination focuses on how internal criticism is delivered, often revealing harsh, contemptuous, or dismissive tones that would be considered abusive if directed toward others. This examination helps members recognize the severity of their self-treatment while building motivation for change.

Trigger identification reveals situations, emotions, or experiences that tend to activate punitive parent voices. Common triggers include mistakes, criticism from others, expressions of need or vulnerability, success or recognition, and interpersonal conflicts.

Historical origins exploration helps members understand where critical voices originated without requiring extensive trauma processing. This understanding reduces the voices' power while helping members recognize that internal criticism reflects past experiences rather than current reality.

Impact assessment examines how punitive parent voices affect daily life, relationships, decision-making, and overall wellbeing. This assessment often reveals that internal criticism creates more problems than it solves while interfering with the very goals it claims to support.

Robert's punitive parent voice delivered relentless criticism about his emotional needs, telling him he was "weak" for needing support, "selfish" for having feelings, and "pathetic" for struggling with trauma symptoms. This voice sounded remarkably similar to his military father, who had taught him that emotions were signs of weakness and that real men handled problems alone.

Through voice identification work, Robert began recognizing when this internal critic became active, usually during moments when he felt vulnerable or needed support from others. The voice's content focused on themes of weakness, self-reliance, and emotional control that reflected his family's military culture rather than realistic expectations for trauma recovery.

Understanding the historical origins of this voice helped Robert recognize that his internal criticism reflected his father's own trauma and emotional limitations rather than accurate assessments of Robert's character or worth. This recognition began creating space between Robert and the critical voice while opening possibilities for developing more compassionate self-talk.

Compassion-Focused Interventions

Compassion-focused therapy approaches, developed by Paul Gilbert (19), provide structured methods for developing self-compassion while addressing the fear and resistance that many trauma survivors experience around treating themselves kindly.

Compassion cultivation exercises help members develop the capacity for self-kindness through practices that gradually build comfort with treating themselves as they would treat beloved friends or family members. These exercises often begin with extending compassion toward others before gradually including oneself.

Self-compassion components include mindfulness (recognizing suffering without over-identification), common humanity (understanding that struggle is part of human experience), and kindness (treating oneself with warmth and understanding). These components work together to create alternatives to self-criticism and shame.

Compassionate self-talk involves developing internal voices that provide support, encouragement, and realistic perspective during difficult times. This compassionate voice serves as an antidote to punitive parent messages while providing internal resources for managing challenges and setbacks.

Loving-kindness meditation practices help members develop genuine feelings of warmth and care toward themselves and others. These practices often begin with easy recipients (beloved pets or children) before gradually including more challenging targets, including oneself.

Compassionate imagery uses visualization to create internal experiences of being cared for, understood, and supported. These imagery practices help members access feelings of safety and acceptance that may have been missing from their actual childhood experiences.

Obstacle identification recognizes that developing self-compassion can feel threatening or dangerous to trauma survivors who learned that self-criticism provided protection against external attack or abandonment. Addressing these obstacles with understanding reduces resistance while maintaining safety.

Jennifer initially struggled with compassion-focused interventions, finding self-kindness "stupid" and "self-indulgent." Her punitive parent voice told her that self-compassion would make her lazy, selfish, and ultimately less successful in life. This resistance reflected childhood experiences where self-care was criticized as selfishness.

The facilitator helped Jennifer experiment with extending compassion toward her resistance rather than fighting it, recognizing that her protective mechanisms had important functions and deserved understanding rather than attack. This approach reduced Jennifer's internal conflict while gradually opening space for self-kindness.

Through group exercises, Jennifer practiced extending compassion toward other members' struggles before gradually applying similar kindness to her own experiences. Witnessing how naturally she offered support and understanding to others helped her recognize the double standard she applied to herself while building confidence in her capacity for compassion.

Reparenting Exercises in Group Context

Reparenting work provides opportunities for group members to offer themselves the care, validation, and support they needed but didn't receive during childhood. This work requires careful facilitation to avoid overwhelming members while creating genuine experiences of being nurtured and valued.

Inner child identification helps members connect with younger versions of themselves who carry wounds from childhood experiences. This identification should be gentle and gradual, respecting members' comfort levels while building relationships with vulnerable internal parts.

Needs assessment explores what inner child parts needed during difficult childhood experiences—safety, validation, protection, comfort, or simply someone who cared about their wellbeing. Understanding these needs provides direction for reparenting work while honoring the reality of what was missing.

Adult resource identification helps members recognize the resources they now possess as adults that weren't available during childhood. These resources might include knowledge, skills, relationships, financial independence, or simply the freedom to make choices about their own lives.

Reparenting visualization provides structured opportunities for members to offer their child selves the care and support they needed, using their adult resources to provide comfort, protection, or validation for past experiences.

Letter writing exercises allow members to communicate with their younger selves through writing, offering wisdom, comfort, and perspective while validating childhood experiences and feelings.

Group reparenting involves other group members offering support and validation to individuals' child parts, providing corrective experiences of being cared for by safe adults who understand trauma's impact.

David's reparenting work focused on providing comfort and protection to his eight-year-old self, who had been terrified and alone after his parents' violent divorce. His inner child carried fear, confusion, and self-blame about the family's dissolution while desperately needing someone to provide reassurance and stability.

Through visualization exercises, David imagined holding his younger self while explaining that the divorce wasn't his fault, that he was loved and valuable, and that he would be okay even though things felt scary and uncertain. This reparenting work helped heal decades of carried fear while providing his inner child with the comfort that had been missing during the actual experience.

The group participated in David's reparenting by offering validation and support to his child self, telling him he deserved safety and love while expressing appreciation for his survival through difficult circumstances. This collective reparenting provided powerful corrective experiences while demonstrating healthy adult care and protection.

Developing Self-Compassion Practices

Building sustainable self-compassion requires ongoing practice as members gradually replace habitual self-criticism with more supportive internal relationships. These practices must be adapted to individual comfort levels while building genuine capacity for self-kindness.

Daily self-compassion check-ins involve brief practices of noticing when members are struggling while offering themselves the same kindness they would extend to good friends facing similar difficulties. These check-ins help build habits of self-support while interrupting automatic self-criticism patterns.

Compassionate self-talk development helps members create specific phrases or statements that provide comfort and support during difficult times. These statements should feel authentic and meaningful rather than empty platitudes while offering genuine alternatives to punitive parent messages.

Self-care practices extend beyond basic physical needs to include emotional, social, and spiritual self-care that honors members' full humanity. These practices should feel nourishing rather than obligatory while building sustainable approaches to self-support and wellbeing.

Mistake and failure processing helps members respond to errors and setbacks with understanding and learning rather than self-attack and shame. This processing recognizes that mistakes are normal parts of human experience while maintaining accountability without self-punishment.

138

Success and achievement integration addresses difficulties that many trauma survivors experience with receiving recognition or feeling proud of accomplishments. Self-compassion includes celebrating successes while avoiding perfectionist standards that make achievement feel hollow or temporary.

Boundary setting support helps members extend compassion to themselves when they need to set limits with others, recognizing that healthy boundaries represent self-care rather than selfishness.

Lisa developed a daily practice of writing brief notes to herself, offering encouragement and support as she would to a dear friend facing similar challenges. These notes helped her recognize her own struggles with compassion while building habits of internal kindness and support.

She also created specific self-talk phrases for common difficult situations—"This is hard, and it makes sense that I'm struggling" for overwhelming moments, "I'm learning and growing, and that's enough" for perceived failures, and "I deserve care and support" when her people-pleasing patterns led to self-neglect.

Through practice, Lisa began noticing when her punitive parent voice became active while having ready alternatives that felt authentic and supportive. This internal shift reduced her anxiety and depression while improving her capacity for healthy relationships and self-advocacy.

Challenging Perfectionist Standards

Perfectionism often masks deep shame, creating impossible standards that guarantee failure while providing evidence for punitive parent attacks. Addressing perfectionism requires understanding its protective functions while developing more realistic and self-compassionate approaches to achievement and growth.

Perfectionism vs. healthy striving helps members distinguish between standards that promote growth and those that create suffering. Healthy striving involves working toward meaningful goals while accepting that mistakes and limitations are normal parts of human experience.

All-or-nothing thinking identification reveals how perfectionist thinking creates false dichotomies where anything less than perfect equals total failure. Challenging this thinking helps members recognize gradations of success while developing more nuanced self-evaluation.

Good enough practices help members experiment with completing tasks or achieving goals without requiring perfection. These experiments often reveal that "good enough" actually produces better results than perfectionist approaches while reducing stress and increasing productivity.

Mistake reframing helps members view errors as learning opportunities rather than evidence of personal inadequacy. This reframing reduces shame while promoting growth and resilience in facing challenges and setbacks.

Realistic standard setting involves establishing goals and expectations that challenge members while remaining achievable. These standards should promote growth while avoiding the paralysis that impossible expectations create.

Process vs. outcome focus shifts attention from perfect results to effort, learning, and growth. This focus reduces anxiety while promoting engagement and persistence in pursuing meaningful goals.

Michael's perfectionism showed up in his work performance, where he spent excessive time on projects trying to achieve impossible standards while criticizing himself harshly for any perceived mistakes or limitations. This pattern created chronic stress while actually reducing his effectiveness and job satisfaction.

Through group work, Michael began experimenting with "good enough" approaches to non-critical tasks while reserving perfectionist energy for truly important projects. He discovered that allowing some

140

projects to be merely adequate actually improved his overall performance by freeing energy for higher-priority work.

The group helped Michael recognize that his perfectionism reflected attempts to avoid criticism and rejection rather than genuine commitment to excellence. Understanding this protective function helped him develop more balanced approaches to achievement while reducing the internal pressure that had been driving his overwork and anxiety.

Integration and Daily Practice

Shame healing requires consistent practice as members gradually replace decades of self-attack with more compassionate internal relationships. Integration work helps members maintain progress while building sustainable approaches to self-compassion and worthiness.

Progress recognition helps members notice positive changes in their self-talk and internal relationships while avoiding perfectionist expectations about shame healing. This recognition builds motivation while acknowledging that healing happens gradually rather than suddenly.

Setback normalization addresses the reality that self-criticism patterns may resurface during stress or difficulty. Normalizing setbacks reduces shame about shame while maintaining commitment to ongoing healing and growth.

Support system utilization helps members identify relationships and resources that support their self-compassion work while providing external validation and encouragement during difficult times.

Environmental assessment examines how members' living and working environments support or undermine their shame healing work while identifying changes that might promote greater self-acceptance and wellbeing.

Meaning-making exploration helps members understand how their shame healing contributes to broader life purposes while connecting self-compassion work to values and goals that extend beyond personal healing.

Legacy considerations explore how members' shame healing affects their relationships with others, particularly children or other vulnerable individuals who might benefit from witnessing healthy self-treatment and compassion.

Sarah's integration work involved creating environmental supports for her self-compassion practice, including posting encouraging notes where she would see them during difficult moments and surrounding herself with images and objects that reminded her of her worth and progress.

She also developed relationships with group members and other supportive people who reinforced her self-compassion work while providing external validation when her internal critic became loud or persistent. These relationships helped sustain her progress while providing models of healthy self-treatment.

Most importantly, Sarah began recognizing how her increased self-compassion affected her relationships with her children, providing them with models of healthy self-treatment while reducing the harsh criticism she had previously modeled. This recognition connected her personal healing to broader purposes while motivating continued growth.

Transformation Through Self-Acceptance

The shame healing work of sessions sixteen through eighteen often creates profound shifts in group members' relationship with themselves and their capacity for authentic connection with others. As self-attack diminishes, energy becomes available for growth, creativity, and genuine intimacy that shame had previously prevented.

Members often discover that they are more likeable, capable, and deserving of love than their shame had convinced them. This discovery doesn't eliminate all self-doubt or difficulty but creates space for self-acceptance that supports continued healing and growth.

The group process itself becomes a laboratory for practicing shame resilience as members experiment with vulnerability, receive support during difficult times, and witness each other's courage in facing internal criticism. These shared experiences create bonds that often extend beyond formal treatment while providing ongoing resources for shame healing.

The internal peace that emerges from reduced self-attack provides foundations for the relationship work that follows, as members become capable of greater intimacy and authenticity when they're not constantly defending against internal criticism and shame.

Core Principles for Healing

- Understanding the distinction between toxic shame and healthy guilt provides frameworks for recognizing and addressing self-attack patterns
- Identifying internalized critical voices helps members recognize punitive parent messages while understanding their historical origins and current impact
- Compassion-focused interventions provide structured approaches for developing self-kindness while addressing resistance and obstacles to self-compassion
- Reparenting exercises offer opportunities to provide inner child parts with the care and validation they needed but didn't receive
- Self-compassion practices build sustainable approaches to internal kindness while replacing habitual self-criticism with supportive self-talk
- Challenging perfectionist standards helps members develop realistic expectations while focusing on growth and learning rather than impossible achievements

Chapter 13: Healing Attachment Wounds and Relational Trauma (Sessions 19-21)

Love feels dangerous when it has been the source of your deepest wounds. For trauma survivors whose injuries occurred within relationships—through childhood abuse, domestic violence, betrayal by trusted others—the very connections they most need for healing can trigger the same nervous system responses that once protected them from harm. Sessions nineteen through twenty-one address this fundamental paradox, helping group members recognize their attachment patterns while gradually building capacity for healthy intimacy and trust.

The group itself becomes the laboratory where these relational experiments unfold. Members practice vulnerability with others who understand trauma's impact, experience corrective relationship dynamics, and develop new templates for what safe connection can look like. This work requires immense courage, as it asks trauma survivors to risk their hearts in service of their healing.

Attachment Styles and Group Dynamics

Attachment patterns formed in our earliest relationships create blueprints for all future connections, influencing how we approach intimacy, handle conflict, and manage the delicate balance between autonomy and connection. Understanding these patterns helps group members recognize their relationship tendencies while developing more conscious choices about how they connect with others.

Secure attachment develops when caregivers consistently respond to children's needs with sensitivity and reliability. Securely attached individuals generally feel comfortable with intimacy and autonomy, communicate their needs directly, and manage relationship conflicts without becoming overwhelmed or shutting down. In group settings, these members often serve as models of healthy relating while providing stability during difficult group dynamics.

144

Anxious attachment emerges when caregivers are inconsistent—sometimes responsive and nurturing, other times distant or rejecting. Anxiously attached individuals often crave closeness while simultaneously fearing abandonment, leading to relationship patterns characterized by clinginess, jealousy, and constant need for reassurance. In groups, these members may monopolize attention, become distressed when others receive focus, or interpret neutral behaviors as signs of rejection.

Avoidant attachment develops when caregivers consistently reject emotional needs or punish expressions of vulnerability. Avoidantly attached individuals learn to suppress their needs for connection while maintaining rigid self-reliance. In group settings, these members may participate intellectually while remaining emotionally distant, resist offers of support, or become uncomfortable when others express strong emotions.

Disorganized attachment results from caregivers who are simultaneously sources of comfort and threat, often due to their own trauma histories or mental health struggles. Individuals with disorganized attachment patterns may display confusing combinations of anxious and avoidant behaviors, rapidly shifting between approach and withdrawal in relationships. Group dynamics with these members can feel unpredictable and intense.

Earned security represents the possibility that individuals can develop secure attachment patterns through healing relationships, even when their early experiences were insecure. Group therapy provides opportunities for earning security through corrective relational experiences with therapists and fellow group members.

Robert's avoidant attachment patterns became evident early in group process as he consistently arrived exactly on time, sat in the same chair near the door, and participated through intellectual analysis rather than emotional sharing. When other members expressed appreciation for him or offered support, he would deflect with humor or minimize the significance of their gestures.

His attachment style made sense given his childhood with emotionally distant parents who valued independence and achievement while discouraging emotional expression or vulnerability. Robert had learned that needing others led to disappointment and that safety came through self-reliance and emotional control.

The group's consistent, non-demanding warmth gradually challenged Robert's avoidant patterns. When Jennifer thanked him for his calming presence during her difficult session, Robert initially deflected but then noticed his automatic response. With group support, he experimented with simply saying "thank you" rather than minimizing the feedback, creating small openings for connection.

Corrective Relational Experiences

The power of group therapy lies partly in its capacity to provide relationship experiences that contradict trauma-based expectations about connection and safety. These corrective experiences don't erase attachment wounds but create new neural pathways that support healthier relating patterns.

Consistent availability of group members and facilitators provides reliability that may have been missing in early relationships. This consistency helps anxiously attached members experience security while helping avoidant members risk gradual connection without fear of sudden abandonment or engulfment.

Attuned responsiveness occurs when group members accurately perceive and respond to each other's emotional states and needs. This attunement helps repair early experiences of misattunement while building capacity for recognizing and meeting others' needs appropriately.

Emotional validation provides acceptance of all emotional experiences without judgment or attempts to fix or change others' feelings. This validation contradicts messages that emotions are wrong, excessive, or dangerous while building tolerance for emotional expression and intimacy.

Conflict repair opportunities arise naturally in group settings, providing chances to experience disagreement or misunderstanding followed by reconnection and resolution. These repair experiences help members learn that relationship ruptures don't necessarily lead to permanent damage or abandonment.

Boundaries and respect demonstrated through group interactions help members experience relationships where individual needs and limits are honored rather than violated or ignored. These experiences provide templates for healthy boundary-setting and respect in other relationships.

Mutual support develops as group members provide care and assistance to each other during difficult times. This reciprocal support helps members experience both giving and receiving care while building confidence in their capacity for healthy interdependence.

Maria's corrective experiences centered around learning that expressing needs didn't lead to punishment or abandonment. Her childhood experiences of sexual abuse had taught her that her needs didn't matter and that speaking up about problems led to blame and further victimization.

When Maria hesitantly shared that she needed more support during her trauma processing work, the group responded with immediate validation and offers of specific help. Rather than being criticized for being "needy" or "dramatic," she experienced her needs being taken seriously and met with compassion.

This experience challenged Maria's core beliefs about relationships while providing a template for healthy need expression and response. Gradually, she began expressing needs more directly in other relationships while developing confidence that appropriate support would be available.

Boundary Setting and Healthy Intimacy

Trauma survivors often struggle with boundaries—either having rigid walls that prevent intimacy or having no boundaries at all, leading to enmeshment and violation. Learning to set and maintain appropriate boundaries becomes essential for developing healthy relationships while protecting against future harm.

Boundary identification helps group members recognize their own needs, preferences, and limits while developing awareness of what feels comfortable versus overwhelming in relationships. This identification process often reveals that members have been ignoring or suppressing their boundary needs to avoid conflict or abandonment.

Types of boundaries include physical boundaries (comfort with touch and personal space), emotional boundaries (what feelings they're willing to share or absorb from others), intellectual boundaries (respecting different opinions), and sexual boundaries (comfort with intimacy and sexual expression).

Boundary communication involves learning to express limits and preferences directly while maintaining respect for others' boundaries. This communication requires balancing assertiveness with empathy while avoiding either aggressive demanding or passive surrender of personal needs.

Boundary enforcement teaches members how to maintain their limits when others push against them, including specific strategies for responding to boundary violations without becoming aggressive or giving in to pressure.

Flexible boundaries help members adjust their level of openness based on relationship context, individual comfort, and specific circumstances. This flexibility prevents both rigid isolation and inappropriate over-sharing while promoting healthy intimacy.

Intimacy gradation involves understanding that healthy relationships involve gradual increases in closeness and vulnerability rather than immediate deep sharing or complete emotional distance. This

148

gradation helps members pace their relationship development appropriately.

Jennifer's boundary work revealed that she had virtually no emotional boundaries, automatically absorbing others' emotions while struggling to identify her own feelings and needs. This pattern had developed as a survival strategy in her chaotic childhood home where monitoring others' emotions was necessary for physical and emotional safety.

Through group exercises, Jennifer practiced identifying her own emotional state before tuning into others' feelings. She learned to ask herself "What am I feeling right now?" before automatically responding to others' emotional expressions, helping her maintain emotional separation while still being responsive and caring.

The group also helped Jennifer practice saying no to requests that felt overwhelming while maintaining connection with the requesting person. These exercises helped her discover that she could set limits without being rejected or abandoned, gradually building confidence in her right to have boundaries.

Trust-Building Exercises and Vulnerability Practices

Trust develops gradually through repeated experiences of safety, reliability, and appropriate response to vulnerability. Group settings provide structured opportunities for trust-building while honoring members' need to proceed at their own pace.

Trust assessment exercises help members identify their current capacity for trust while recognizing how trauma may have affected their ability to discern trustworthy individuals and situations. This assessment includes understanding the difference between healthy caution and trauma-based hypervigilance.

Graduated vulnerability involves sharing increasingly personal information over time while gauging others' responses and adjusting based on feedback. This graduated approach prevents overwhelming

149

exposure while building confidence in both sharing and receiving vulnerable information.

Reciprocal sharing creates opportunities for mutual vulnerability where group members take turns sharing personal experiences while supporting each other through the disclosure process. This reciprocity helps balance giving and receiving while building mutual trust and understanding.

Trust repair exercises address situations where trust has been damaged through misunderstanding, boundary violations, or insensitive responses. These exercises help members learn that trust can be rebuilt after ruptures while developing skills for repair processes.

Risk assessment skills help members evaluate potential relationships and situations for trustworthiness while avoiding both excessive caution that prevents connection and naive trust that ignores warning signs.

Self-trust development focuses on building confidence in members' own perceptions, feelings, and judgments about relationships and situations. Trauma often damages self-trust, leading individuals to doubt their own assessments while relying excessively on others' opinions.

David's trust-building work focused on his tendency to either trust completely or not at all, reflecting his disorganized attachment patterns from childhood. He would often share very personal information early in relationships while simultaneously remaining suspicious of others' motives and responses.

Through group exercises, David practiced sharing moderately personal information while paying attention to how others responded. He learned to look for signs of genuine interest, appropriate boundaries, and emotional safety rather than just reciprocal disclosure or dramatic reactions.

The group helped David recognize that healthy trust develops through consistent small interactions rather than dramatic gestures or immediate deep connection. This understanding helped him develop more realistic expectations for relationship development while reducing his tendency toward intense, unstable connections.

Addressing Betrayal Trauma and Relationship Fears

Betrayal trauma—harm inflicted by individuals who were supposed to provide care and protection—creates particularly complex relationship challenges. Survivors must heal from specific traumatic experiences while rebuilding their capacity to trust and connect with others.

Betrayal trauma identification helps members recognize how violations by trusted others affect their current relationship patterns and fears. This identification includes understanding how betrayal trauma differs from other trauma types in its impact on trust, attachment, and relationship expectations.

Fear exploration examines specific relationship fears that stem from betrayal experiences, such as fear of abandonment, fear of engulfment, fear of rejection, or fear of further betrayal. Understanding these fears helps members respond to them consciously rather than being controlled by unconscious avoidance patterns.

Safety signal development helps members identify signs that relationships are likely to be safe and trustworthy while developing skills for recognizing potential dangers or red flags. This development balances appropriate caution with openness to connection.

Trauma timeline processing may involve exploring how betrayal experiences affect current relationship patterns without requiring detailed trauma processing. This exploration helps members understand their reactions while maintaining focus on current relationship development.

Relationship pattern recognition helps members identify recurring dynamics in their relationships that may reflect unresolved betrayal trauma, such as choosing untrustworthy partners, sabotaging healthy relationships, or remaining in harmful connections.

Protective factor strengthening involves building internal and external resources that support relationship safety while reducing vulnerability to future betrayal or harm.

Lisa's betrayal trauma from childhood sexual abuse by a family friend created complex fears about trusting her own judgment in relationships. She had learned to ignore her intuitive concerns about people while focusing exclusively on others' needs and presentations of themselves.

Through group work, Lisa began reconnecting with her internal warning systems while learning to trust her gut feelings about people and situations. The group helped her recognize that her intuition had actually been quite accurate but that she had learned to discount it in favor of others' reassurances or explanations.

This work helped Lisa develop confidence in her ability to assess relationship safety while reducing her tendency to remain in harmful or unfulfilling connections out of fear, guilt, or misplaced loyalty.

Practicing Healthy Relationships in the Group

The group becomes a real-time laboratory for practicing healthier relationship patterns while receiving immediate feedback about interpersonal impact and effectiveness. These practice opportunities provide safe contexts for experimenting with new ways of relating.

Communication skill practice involves experimenting with direct, honest communication while learning to express needs, feelings, and concerns in ways that promote understanding rather than conflict or withdrawal.

Conflict resolution opportunities arise naturally in group settings, providing chances to practice navigating disagreements while maintaining respect and connection. These practices help members learn that conflict doesn't necessarily damage relationships when handled skillfully.

Support giving and receiving helps members practice both offering appropriate help to others and accepting support when they need it. These practices address common trauma-related difficulties with interdependence and reciprocity.

Emotional regulation in relationships involves managing intense emotions during interpersonal interactions while maintaining connection and appropriate expression. This regulation helps prevent relationship damage from emotional overwhelm or shutdown.

Authenticity practice encourages members to be genuine in their group interactions while maintaining appropriate boundaries and consideration for others. This authenticity helps members experience being loved for who they truly are rather than who they think they should be.

Intimacy tolerance building helps members gradually increase their comfort with emotional closeness while maintaining individual identity and autonomy. This building helps prevent both isolation and enmeshment in relationships.

Michael's relationship practice in the group focused on his tendency to withdraw emotionally when conflicts arose, a pattern that had damaged his marriage and other important relationships. With group support, he began practicing staying present during disagreements while expressing his perspective directly.

During one group session, Michael disagreed with another member's interpretation of his behavior, feeling criticized and misunderstood. Rather than his usual pattern of shutting down or leaving, he practiced expressing his feelings while remaining open to the other person's perspective.

This practice helped Michael discover that he could maintain connection during conflict while still protecting his own needs and boundaries. The successful navigation of this disagreement provided a template he could apply to conflicts with his wife and other important relationships.

Building Secure Relationships

The ultimate goal of attachment healing work involves developing the capacity for secure relationships characterized by appropriate intimacy, effective communication, mutual support, and resilience in facing challenges together.

Secure relationship characteristics include comfort with both closeness and independence, ability to communicate needs and feelings directly, capacity for conflict resolution without relationship threat, and mutual support during difficulties and celebrations.

Internal security development involves building self-worth and emotional regulation that doesn't depend entirely on relationship status or others' approval. This internal security provides the foundation for healthy relationships while preventing codependence or desperate attachment.

Relationship selection skills help members choose partners and friends who are capable of healthy relating while avoiding individuals who are likely to recreate traumatic relationship patterns.

Maintenance strategies provide ongoing approaches for nurturing healthy relationships while addressing inevitable challenges and changes that occur over time.

Generational healing explores how members' relationship healing affects their children, family members, and community, potentially breaking cycles of trauma and unhealthy relating patterns.

Sarah's secure relationship development involved learning to balance her strong caretaking tendencies with appropriate attention to her own needs and boundaries. Through group work, she practiced being supportive without becoming responsible for others' emotions or problems.

She also learned to receive support from others without feeling guilty or burdensome, gradually building confidence that she deserved care and that healthy relationships involved mutual giving and receiving rather than one-sided caretaking.

These changes in Sarah's group relationships translated into improvements in her marriage and friendships, as she became more authentic and balanced in her connections while maintaining her naturally caring personality.

The Courage to Love Again

Healing attachment wounds requires extraordinary courage—the willingness to risk rejection, disappointment, or even retraumatization in service of the human need for connection and love. Group members who engage in this work demonstrate remarkable bravery while supporting each other through the vulnerable process of opening their hearts again.

The relationships formed during group treatment often become templates for future connections while providing ongoing sources of support and validation. Members learn through direct experience that healthy relationships are possible while developing skills and confidence for creating such relationships in their broader lives.

The attachment healing that occurs in group settings often extends far beyond the treatment room, affecting members' relationships with partners, children, friends, and colleagues. This ripple effect demonstrates the profound impact that healing core relationship wounds can have on all aspects of life and wellbeing.

Relationship Foundations

- Understanding attachment styles helps members recognize their relationship patterns while developing more conscious choices about how they connect with others
- Corrective relational experiences within the group contradict trauma-based expectations while creating new templates for healthy connection and intimacy
- Boundary setting and healthy intimacy skills help members balance closeness and autonomy while protecting against violation and maintaining authentic connection
- Trust-building exercises provide graduated approaches to vulnerability while developing skills for assessing relationship safety and trustworthiness
- Addressing betrayal trauma helps members process specific relationship wounds while rebuilding capacity for trust and connection with others
- Practicing healthy relationships in the group provides real-time opportunities for developing secure relating patterns while receiving immediate feedback and support

Chapter 14: Working with Dissociation and Parts (Sessions 22-24)

Dissociation whispers its protection: "You don't have to be here for this." In moments of overwhelming threat or unbearable pain, the mind's capacity to disconnect from present experience becomes a lifesaving gift. But what serves as protection during trauma can become a prison in safety, leaving individuals feeling fragmented, unreal, or absent from their own lives. Sessions twenty-two through twenty-four address dissociation's complex nature, helping group members understand their disconnection patterns while building capacity for grounded, integrated presence.

This work requires extraordinary sensitivity, as pushing too quickly toward integration can trigger the very overwhelm that dissociation protects against. Yet with careful pacing and skilled support, group members can learn to appreciate their mind's protective wisdom while developing choice about when and how to be present in their experience.

Dissociation Assessment and Mapping

Understanding dissociation begins with recognizing its many forms, from mild spacing out during stressful conversations to complete amnesia for traumatic events. Assessment helps group members identify their unique dissociation patterns while developing language for describing experiences that often feel impossible to put into words.

Types of dissociation range along a continuum from normal to pathological responses. Mild dissociation includes daydreaming, highway hypnosis, or becoming absorbed in activities to the point of losing track of time. Moderate dissociation involves feeling unreal, watching oneself from outside, or experiencing emotional numbness during stressful events. Severe dissociation includes amnesia, identity confusion, or complete disconnection from physical sensations and emotional experiences.

Dissociation triggers often relate to specific situations, emotions, or sensations that activate protective disconnection responses. Common triggers include conflict, criticism, intimacy, medical procedures, anniversary dates, or any situation that resembles aspects of original traumatic experiences.

Dissociation mapping creates visual or descriptive representations of individual dissociation patterns, helping members understand when, where, and how they disconnect while identifying what circumstances support presence and integration.

Somatic indicators of dissociation include feeling floaty or ungrounded, numbness or tingling sensations, feeling like the body belongs to someone else, or experiencing physical sensations as distant or muffled. These bodily signs often provide early warning systems for impending dissociation.

Cognitive signs include feeling confused or foggy, difficulty concentrating, memory problems, feeling like thoughts belong to someone else, or experiencing internal dialogue as voices rather than personal thoughts.

Emotional indicators involve feeling numb or empty, experiencing emotions as distant or belonging to others, rapid mood shifts that don't make sense, or feeling like emotional reactions are watching from outside rather than being personally experienced.

Jennifer's dissociation assessment revealed a complex pattern of disconnection that had protected her during childhood sexual abuse but now interfered with her ability to be present in her adult relationships. She identified several specific triggers: being touched unexpectedly, hearing raised voices, medical appointments, and moments of physical intimacy with her husband.

Her dissociation typically began with a floating sensation, as if she were rising above her body to observe from the ceiling. During these episodes, she could see and hear what was happening but felt no emotional connection to the events. Sometimes she would lose time completely, finding herself in different locations with no memory of how she got there.

Through mapping exercises, Jennifer began recognizing early warning signs of impending dissociation, including shallow breathing, feeling cold, and a sense of everything becoming distant or unreal. This awareness provided opportunities for intervention before complete disconnection occurred.

Grounding Techniques for Dissociative Episodes

Grounding interventions help bring consciousness back into the body and present moment, countering dissociation's disconnection through sensory anchoring and present-moment awareness. These techniques must be adapted for individuals whose nervous systems may be hypersensitive to certain sensory inputs.

Sensory grounding uses multiple senses to anchor awareness in current reality. The 5-4-3-2-1 technique involves identifying five things you can see, four things you can touch, three things you can hear, two things you can smell, and one thing you can taste. This systematic sensory engagement helps reconnect with immediate environmental reality.

Physical grounding uses direct contact with solid surfaces or objects to help individuals feel more present in their bodies. This might include pressing feet firmly into the floor, placing hands on walls or furniture, holding textured objects, or using weighted blankets or lap pads.

Movement grounding employs gentle physical activity to reconnect with bodily sensations and present-moment awareness. Simple movements like stretching, walking, or bilateral activities (alternating left and right movements) can help reintegrate consciousness with physical experience.

Breathing anchors use focused attention on breath to ground awareness in the body. However, breath-focused techniques must be used carefully with trauma survivors, as some individuals find breath focus triggering rather than grounding.

Environmental grounding helps individuals connect with their immediate surroundings through detailed observation and interaction. This might involve naming objects in the room, identifying colors and textures, or engaging with environmental features like temperature or lighting.

Interpersonal grounding uses connection with others to anchor present-moment awareness. This might include making eye contact with supportive others, hearing familiar voices, or receiving appropriate physical contact from trusted individuals.

When Robert noticed Jennifer beginning to dissociate during a group session—her eyes becoming unfocused and her body very still—he gently said her name and asked if she could feel her feet on the floor. The facilitator guided Jennifer through a brief grounding sequence, asking her to name three things she could see in the room, then to press her hands firmly against her legs.

This intervention helped Jennifer return to present-moment awareness without feeling criticized or abnormal for her dissociative response. The group's calm, supportive handling of her dissociation helped normalize this protective mechanism while demonstrating that others could help her stay present when needed.

Over time, Jennifer developed her own grounding toolkit, including a small stone she carried for tactile grounding, peppermint oil for scent anchoring, and specific phrases she could repeat to help her stay connected to current reality.

Parts Work with Dissociative Clients

Dissociation often reflects the activity of protective parts that remove consciousness from overwhelming situations. Working with these parts requires understanding their protective functions while gradually building safety and capacity for more integrated awareness.

Protector parts identification helps recognize aspects of the personality that create dissociative responses to protect against overwhelming experiences. These parts often carry important information about what feels dangerous while maintaining responsibility for psychological and sometimes physical survival.

Exile parts recognition involves identifying wounded aspects of the self that dissociative protectors are trying to shield from further harm. These exiled parts often carry traumatic memories, intense emotions, or experiences that feel too overwhelming to integrate fully.

Firefighter parts may create dissociation to escape unbearable internal states, using disconnection as a form of relief from overwhelming emotions or sensations. Understanding these parts helps reduce judgment about dissociative responses while addressing underlying needs for comfort and safety.

Internal negotiation with dissociative parts involves respectful dialogue about their protective functions while exploring possibilities for maintaining safety without complete disconnection. This negotiation requires patience and genuine appreciation for parts' protective efforts.

Safety building for dissociative parts includes creating internal and external conditions that support their gradual trust in present-moment safety. This safety building often requires addressing current life circumstances that may continue triggering protective disconnection.

Integration support helps dissociative parts gradually allow more presence and connection while maintaining their protective capacity when genuinely needed. Integration doesn't eliminate dissociative capacity but creates choice about when and how to use this protective mechanism.

Maria's parts work revealed a young protector part that created dissociation whenever she felt trapped or powerless, removing her consciousness from situations that resembled her childhood abuse experiences. This part had likely saved her sanity during repeated traumatic events but now activated during normal relationship conflicts or even routine medical appointments.

Through gentle dialogue, Maria learned to appreciate this protector's life-saving service while helping it recognize that she now had adult resources for handling difficult situations. The protector part gradually learned to trust Maria's ability to protect herself while maintaining its readiness to provide dissociative protection if truly needed.

This internal negotiation reduced Maria's automatic dissociation while maintaining access to protective disconnection during genuinely overwhelming situations. The result was greater presence in daily life while preserving important protective capacities.

Group Containment and Safety Protocols

Working with dissociation in group settings requires sophisticated safety protocols that protect dissociating individuals while maintaining group stability and safety for all members. These protocols must address the reality that dissociation can be contagious, triggering similar responses in other trauma survivors.

Dissociation recognition training helps group members and facilitators identify signs of dissociation in themselves and others while developing appropriate responses that support rather than increase disconnection.

Intervention protocols establish clear procedures for responding when group members dissociate, including immediate safety assessment, grounding support, and decisions about whether to continue group activities or provide individual attention.

Contagion prevention addresses the reality that one person's dissociation can trigger similar responses in other group members, requiring interventions that support the dissociating individual while maintaining group stability.

Safety anchoring involves maintaining consistent environmental and interpersonal cues that support present-moment awareness while reducing triggers that might activate dissociative responses.

Co-regulation support uses the nervous systems of non-dissociated group members and facilitators to help support the regulation of individuals who have disconnected from their own bodily awareness.

Integration pacing ensures that work with dissociation proceeds at appropriate speeds that build capacity without overwhelming individuals or triggering increased fragmentation.

During one group session, David began dissociating while listening to another member process childhood abuse memories. His dissociation triggered similar responses in two other members, creating a group dynamic where several people were disconnected from present-moment awareness.

The facilitator immediately implemented safety protocols, first ensuring that all members were physically safe, then providing individual grounding support to help each person return to present awareness. The session focus shifted from trauma processing to present-moment stabilization until all members felt grounded and connected.

This experience led to enhanced group protocols for managing dissociation, including buddy systems where members could support each other's grounding and agreements about how to handle situations where multiple members became dissociated simultaneously.

Integration and Co-Consciousness Development

The goal of dissociation work isn't to eliminate protective disconnection but to develop choice and awareness about when dissociation occurs while building capacity for integrated consciousness during safe situations.

Awareness building helps individuals recognize when they're beginning to dissociate while developing skills for conscious choice about whether to continue the disconnection or attempt to stay present.

Partial presence practices teach individuals how to maintain some connection to present-moment awareness even when using dissociative protection, creating bridges between full presence and complete disconnection.

Co-consciousness development involves building capacity for different parts of the self to be aware simultaneously rather than requiring complete switching between different states of consciousness.

Memory bridge building helps individuals maintain continuity of experience even when dissociation occurs, reducing amnesia and confusion that can result from complete disconnection.

Integration skills support individuals in gradually increasing their window of tolerance for present-moment experience while maintaining access to protective dissociation when genuinely needed.

Daily life application helps individuals use their developing dissociation awareness and choice in their ongoing lives outside of group sessions.

Lisa's integration work focused on developing what she called "one foot in, one foot out"—maintaining some present-moment awareness even when using dissociative protection during medical procedures that triggered her trauma history.

Through practice, she learned to keep part of her consciousness anchored in current reality (noticing the kind voice of her current doctor, feeling the comfortable temperature of the room) while allowing other parts to disconnect from overwhelming sensations or memories.

This partial presence approach reduced her post-medical appointment confusion and distress while maintaining protective capacity during genuinely difficult procedures. She felt more empowered and less fragmented in her daily life while preserving important protective mechanisms.

Advanced Dissociation Work

As group members develop basic dissociation awareness and management skills, more sophisticated approaches become available for addressing complex dissociative presentations and building greater integration.

Trauma processing with dissociation requires specialized techniques that honor protective disconnection while gradually building capacity for processing traumatic material without complete fragmentation.

Somatic integration helps individuals reconnect with bodily sensations and experiences that may have been dissociated during traumatic events, building bridges between mind and body awareness.

Attachment and dissociation addresses how disconnection affects relationship capacity while building skills for maintaining connection with others even during dissociative episodes.

Identity integration works with individuals who have complex dissociative presentations involving different aspects of identity or personality, supporting cooperation and communication between different parts.

Creativity and dissociation uses artistic expression, movement, and other creative modalities to support integration while honoring the adaptive creativity that dissociation represents.

Spiritual dimensions may address how dissociation affects individuals' sense of meaning, purpose, and connection to something larger than themselves while supporting integration of spiritual resources.

Robert's advanced dissociation work involved processing combat memories that had been completely disconnected from his conscious awareness for years. Through careful, gradual work with group support, he began accessing fragmented memories while maintaining enough present-moment awareness to avoid becoming completely overwhelmed.

This trauma processing work required sophisticated integration of grounding techniques, parts work, and present-moment anchoring while honoring his protective dissociation when the material became too intense to process safely.

The group's witnessing and support provided crucial co-regulation during this advanced work while offering validation for both Robert's traumatic experiences and his mind's protective responses to overwhelming events.

Honoring Protective Wisdom

Working with dissociation requires profound respect for the mind's protective wisdom while supporting individuals in developing greater choice and integration. Dissociation represents one of the most sophisticated protective mechanisms available to human consciousness, often making survival possible in situations that would otherwise be psychologically lethal.

The goal is never to eliminate dissociative capacity but to develop conscious relationship with this protective mechanism while building tolerance for present-moment experience during safe situations. This approach honors trauma survivors' resourcefulness while supporting their capacity for integrated living.

Group work with dissociation often creates powerful healing experiences as members witness each other's courage in facing fragmentation while providing mutual support for integration efforts.

These shared experiences reduce shame about dissociative responses while building community around complex trauma recovery.

The integration work that occurs during these sessions provides foundations for ongoing healing while building skills that members can use throughout their lives to manage dissociation consciously and effectively.

Essential Understanding Points

- Dissociation assessment and mapping help members identify their unique disconnection patterns while developing language for describing complex internal experiences
- Grounding techniques provide concrete tools for returning to present-moment awareness while respecting the protective functions of dissociative responses
- Parts work with dissociative clients requires understanding protective functions while building safety and capacity for more integrated awareness
- Group containment protocols ensure safety for dissociating individuals while preventing contagion and maintaining group stability during difficult work
- Integration and co-consciousness development build choice and awareness about dissociation while maintaining access to protective disconnection when needed
- Advanced techniques address complex dissociative presentations while supporting greater integration and capacity for processing traumatic material safely

Chapter 15: Managing Crisis and Dysregulation in Groups

Crisis doesn't knock before entering the therapy room—it bursts through doors, disrupts carefully planned sessions, and demands immediate, skilled response from facilitators who must balance individual safety with group stability. The moment when a group member becomes suicidal, threatens self-harm, or experiences complete emotional dysregulation tests every aspect of your clinical training while the eyes of seven other trauma survivors watch to see if you can handle what feels unmanageable to them.

These moments separate competent group facilitators from those who should stick to individual work. Crisis management in groups requires split-second decision-making, clear protocols, and the ability to provide life-saving intervention while maintaining therapeutic relationships with multiple people simultaneously. Get it right, and the group becomes stronger. Get it wrong, and you risk losing not just the member in crisis but the trust and safety of everyone else in the room.

Crisis Assessment and Intervention Protocols

Crisis assessment in group settings demands rapid evaluation of multiple factors simultaneously—the immediate safety of the person in crisis, the impact on other group members, available resources, and legal obligations. This assessment must occur while maintaining calm leadership that models effective crisis management for group members who may never have witnessed healthy responses to psychological emergencies.

Immediate safety assessment forms the foundation of all crisis intervention. You must quickly determine if the person presents imminent danger to themselves or others while gathering enough information to make informed decisions about intervention level. This assessment includes evaluating suicide risk, self-harm potential, risk of violence toward others, and capacity for self-care and decision-making.

Risk factors identification helps determine crisis severity and appropriate response level. High-risk factors include specific suicide plans with available means, history of serious suicide attempts, current substance use, social isolation, recent major losses, and presence of psychotic symptoms or severe depression. Medium-risk factors might include passive suicidal ideation, self-harm without suicidal intent, increased substance use, or significant life stressors without adequate support.

Protective factors assessment identifies resources that support safety and recovery. These might include strong therapeutic relationships, family support, religious or spiritual beliefs, future-oriented plans, previous successful crisis management, and access to mental health services. Understanding protective factors helps determine whether outpatient crisis management is appropriate or if higher levels of care are needed.

Group impact evaluation considers how the crisis affects other group members while determining what interventions support both the person in crisis and group stability. Some crises can be managed within the group setting with benefit to all members, while others require removing the individual from the group to prevent destabilization or secondary trauma to other participants.

During a group session, Maria began crying uncontrollably while describing recent flashbacks of childhood sexual abuse. Her crying escalated to hyperventilation and then to statements like "I can't do this anymore" and "I just want it all to stop." The facilitator immediately implemented crisis assessment protocols while maintaining awareness of how other group members were responding to Maria's distress.

The facilitator's rapid assessment revealed that Maria was experiencing intense emotional pain but had no specific plans for suicide or self-harm. She had strong protective factors including her children, her faith, and her commitment to therapy. However, her level of distress was affecting other group members, with two others beginning to dissociate and one becoming agitated.

The intervention involved providing immediate emotional support to Maria while helping her access grounding techniques, briefly checking with other group members about their ability to continue, and making an individual safety assessment before the session ended. This crisis actually strengthened group bonds as members witnessed both Maria's courage in facing her pain and the facilitator's competent response to crisis.

De-escalation Techniques for Group Settings

De-escalation in groups requires managing multiple emotional systems simultaneously while preventing crisis contagion that can destabilize the entire group. Effective de-escalation calms the individual in crisis while modeling emotional regulation for other group members who may struggle with similar issues.

Voice and tone modulation becomes your primary tool for influencing group emotional climate. A calm, steady voice can help regulate not just the person in crisis but the entire group's nervous system. Avoid matching the intensity of the person in crisis, as this can escalate rather than calm the situation.

Active listening and validation help the person in crisis feel heard and understood while demonstrating healthy responses to emotional distress for other group members. This validation doesn't mean agreeing with distorted thinking but acknowledging the person's emotional experience and pain.

Collaborative problem-solving engages the person in crisis as an active participant in their own safety planning rather than imposing solutions. This approach maintains dignity and autonomy while building skills for future crisis management.

Grounding and regulation techniques help return the person to their window of tolerance while teaching other group members concrete skills for managing their own dysregulation. These techniques might include breathing exercises, progressive muscle relaxation, or sensory grounding approaches.

Group support mobilization harnesses the collective wisdom and caring of group members to support the person in crisis while building group cohesion and mutual aid skills. This support must be facilitated carefully to avoid overwhelming the person in crisis or triggering other members.

Robert became increasingly agitated during a group session when discussing his anger toward his ex-wife. His voice became louder, his posture more rigid, and he began making statements about wanting to "teach her a lesson." Other group members became visibly uncomfortable, with some moving their chairs back and others looking toward the door.

The facilitator used de-escalation techniques by first lowering her own voice and speaking more slowly, which naturally encouraged Robert to match her tone. She validated his frustration while redirecting his focus from his ex-wife to his own experience in the moment. "Robert, I can see how angry you're feeling right now. What's happening in your body as you talk about this?"

This intervention helped Robert shift from external blame to internal awareness, reducing his agitation while modeling emotional regulation for other group members. The facilitator then engaged the group in discussing healthy ways to handle anger, turning the crisis into a learning opportunity for everyone.

Suicidal Ideation and Self-Harm Management

Suicidal ideation in group settings creates complex dynamics requiring immediate safety assessment while maintaining therapeutic relationships with multiple group members. The response must balance individual crisis intervention with group stability while meeting legal and ethical obligations for suicide prevention.

Suicide risk assessment must be thorough yet conducted efficiently to minimize group disruption while ensuring safety. This assessment includes evaluating current suicidal thoughts, specific plans, access to means, intent to act, and timeline for potential action. You must also assess protective factors, support systems, and previous suicide attempts or self-harm behaviors.

Immediate safety planning involves collaborating with the person to develop concrete strategies for maintaining safety between sessions and accessing help when needed. Safety plans should be specific, realistic, and include multiple options for support and intervention.

Group disclosure decisions require careful consideration of what information to share with other group members while maintaining confidentiality and therapeutic relationships. Generally, you can acknowledge that someone is struggling without sharing specific details of suicidal thoughts or plans.

Individual attention balance means providing necessary crisis intervention without abandoning other group members or allowing one person's crisis to dominate every session. This might require individual time after group sessions or additional individual appointments between group meetings.

Follow-up protocols ensure ongoing safety monitoring while maintaining group participation when appropriate. This includes clear communication about what will happen next, who will be contacted, and how the person can access support before the next group session.

Jennifer disclosed passive suicidal ideation during a group session, stating that she had been thinking about death frequently and sometimes wished she could just "go to sleep and not wake up." She denied having specific plans but acknowledged feeling hopeless about her ability to recover from trauma.

The facilitator conducted a more detailed risk assessment privately with Jennifer after the group session while arranging for other members to process their reactions to her disclosure. The assessment revealed that Jennifer had no specific plans, no access to lethal means, and strong protective factors including her children and her commitment to therapy.

The safety plan included Jennifer contacting the crisis hotline if thoughts became more specific, checking in with her individual therapist before the next group session, and using group members as support contacts if she felt comfortable doing so. The group became a source of support rather than a burden, with members expressing appreciation for Jennifer's honesty and offering their own experiences of working through suicidal thoughts.

Legal and Ethical Guidelines for Breaking Confidentiality

Group facilitators must navigate complex legal and ethical requirements around confidentiality while managing crisis situations that may require sharing information with outside parties. Understanding these requirements protects both clients and therapists while ensuring appropriate response to genuine safety concerns.

Duty to warn obligations vary by state but generally require therapists to take reasonable steps to protect identifiable third parties when clients make credible threats of violence. In group settings, this might involve other group members, family members, or individuals mentioned during sessions.

Mandatory reporting requirements include situations involving child abuse, elder abuse, or abuse of dependent adults. Group members may disclose information that triggers reporting obligations, requiring therapists to balance confidentiality with legal requirements for protection of vulnerable individuals.

Involuntary commitment procedures become necessary when individuals present imminent danger to themselves or others and lack capacity to make informed decisions about their safety. These procedures vary by jurisdiction but typically require specific documentation and legal processes.

Documentation requirements include detailed records of crisis assessment, interventions provided, safety planning, and follow-up actions taken. This documentation protects both clients and therapists while providing necessary information for ongoing care coordination.

Group member notification may be necessary when confidentiality must be broken, requiring careful communication about what information can be shared and what must remain confidential. Group members need to understand the limits of confidentiality while maintaining trust in the therapeutic process.

During a group session, David disclosed that he had been having detailed fantasies about harming his ex-wife's new boyfriend, including plans for how he would approach the person and what weapons he might use. He stated that he probably wouldn't act on these thoughts but acknowledged feeling increasingly obsessed with the idea.

The facilitator recognized this as a potential duty to warn situation, requiring her to assess the credibility of the threat and take appropriate protective action. After the group session, she conducted a more thorough assessment with David, determining that while his thoughts were detailed, he had no actual intent to harm the individual and recognized that his fantasies were problematic.

The intervention included safety planning with David, coordination with his individual therapist, and consultation with legal experts about duty to warn requirements. No warning was ultimately required because David had no genuine intent to harm, but the facilitator documented the assessment process and safety planning thoroughly.

Emergency Procedures and Aftercare Planning

Emergency procedures in group settings require clear protocols that can be implemented quickly while maintaining safety for all participants. These procedures must address various crisis types while providing frameworks for decision-making under pressure.

Emergency contact protocols ensure that appropriate individuals can be reached quickly when crises occur. This includes emergency contacts for group members, consultation resources for therapists, and crisis intervention services available in the community.

Crisis intervention resources should be readily available and familiar to both facilitators and group members. These might include crisis hotlines, mobile crisis teams, emergency psychiatric services, and immediate psychiatric hospitalization resources.

Group session management during crises requires decisions about continuing sessions, dismissing other members, or modifying group activities based on the severity of the situation. Clear protocols help facilitators make these decisions quickly while maintaining safety and therapeutic relationships.

Individual member support ensures that people in crisis receive appropriate follow-up care while other group members get necessary support for their reactions to crisis events. This might include individual sessions, referrals to additional services, or modifications to group participation.

Documentation and communication requirements include detailed records of crisis events, interventions provided, and outcomes achieved. This documentation supports ongoing care coordination while meeting legal and professional requirements.

Return to group planning helps determine when and how individuals can resume group participation after crisis events, ensuring both individual readiness and group safety and stability.

Lisa experienced a panic attack during group that escalated to thoughts of self-harm, requiring immediate intervention and emergency planning. The facilitator implemented crisis protocols by first ensuring Lisa's immediate safety, then arranging for other group members to be dismissed early with appropriate support and follow-up.

The emergency intervention included a detailed safety assessment, development of an immediate safety plan, coordination with Lisa's individual therapist, and arrangement for Lisa to be driven home by a friend rather than driving herself. The facilitator also contacted Lisa later that evening to check on her status and confirm that she was following through with safety plan elements.

The aftercare planning included an individual session before the next group meeting to process the crisis event and determine readiness to return to group. Lisa was able to resume group participation the following week, and the group processed the experience together, which actually strengthened group bonds and demonstrated effective crisis management.

Crisis Prevention and Early Intervention

While crises can't always be prevented, many can be anticipated and addressed before they reach emergency levels. Effective prevention involves recognizing early warning signs while building group culture that supports help-seeking and mutual support.

Warning sign identification helps both facilitators and group members recognize when someone is approaching crisis levels. These signs might include increased irritability, social withdrawal, changes in appearance or hygiene, increased substance use, or expressions of hopelessness or despair.

Check-in procedures at the beginning of each session provide opportunities for members to report concerns about themselves or others while accessing support before problems escalate to crisis levels.

Peer support systems within the group create networks of mutual monitoring and assistance that can provide early intervention when someone is struggling. These systems must be structured carefully to avoid inappropriate responsibility or codependent dynamics.

Individual attention between sessions may be necessary for group members who are experiencing increased stress or trauma symptoms that could escalate to crisis levels. This might include brief phone calls, email check-ins, or additional individual sessions.

Environmental modifications can reduce crisis risk by addressing factors in group members' lives that contribute to instability. This might include referrals for housing assistance, job placement services, or financial counseling.

Michael's early warning signs included increased tardiness to group sessions, decreased participation in discussions, and subtle expressions of hopelessness about his recovery progress. The facilitator recognized these changes and provided individual attention to assess Michael's status and provide additional support.

The early intervention prevented what could have become a crisis by addressing Michael's growing depression and social withdrawal before they led to suicidal ideation or other dangerous behaviors. The group also participated in supporting Michael, with other members sharing their own experiences of recovery setbacks and offering encouragement and practical support.

This prevention approach reduced the likelihood of crisis while building group cohesion and mutual support skills that benefited all members. Michael was able to work through his difficult period with group support rather than requiring crisis intervention or higher levels of care.

Building Crisis Resilience

The ultimate goal of crisis management in groups is building resilience and skills that help members manage future crises independently while maintaining connection to supportive resources. This resilience building occurs through modeling, skill development, and confidence building during actual crisis events.

Crisis skills development helps group members learn concrete techniques for managing their own crisis situations while supporting others who are struggling. These skills include safety planning, help-seeking, emotional regulation, and social support utilization.

Confidence building occurs as group members witness effective crisis management and participate in supporting others through difficult times. These experiences build confidence in both individual and collective abilities to handle crises effectively.

Resource identification helps group members develop awareness of available crisis resources while building skills for accessing help when needed. This includes professional resources, peer support, family support, and community resources.

Recovery planning from crisis events helps individuals and groups learn from crisis experiences while building stronger prevention and intervention capabilities for the future.

Sarah's crisis resilience developed through her experiences of both receiving and providing crisis support within the group. After working through her own suicidal crisis with group support, she became particularly skilled at recognizing when other members were struggling and offering appropriate assistance.

Her confidence in handling crisis situations grew through these experiences, and she developed a strong network of support resources that included both professional services and peer relationships from the group. This resilience served her well in managing future challenges while maintaining her recovery progress.

The group as a whole became more resilient through their collective experiences of managing crises effectively. Members developed strong mutual support skills while building confidence in their individual and collective abilities to handle difficult situations.

Wisdom Through Crisis

Crisis management in groups tests every aspect of clinical skill while providing opportunities for profound growth and learning. Group members who successfully navigate crises together often develop bonds and skills that serve them throughout their recovery journeys while building confidence in their ability to handle life's challenges.

The key lies in maintaining calm leadership while implementing clear protocols that protect individual safety and group stability. Crisis events, when handled skillfully, can actually strengthen groups and build resilience rather than causing damage or instability.

Effective crisis management requires ongoing training, consultation, and self-care to maintain the skills and emotional resources needed to respond effectively under pressure. The responsibility of managing crisis in groups should not be undertaken lightly, but with proper preparation and support, it becomes one of the most rewarding aspects of group facilitation.

Essential Skills and Knowledge

- Crisis assessment protocols enable rapid evaluation of safety risks while considering impacts on individual group members and overall group stability
- De-escalation techniques help calm individuals in crisis while modeling emotional regulation skills for other group members
- Suicidal ideation management requires thorough risk assessment, safety planning, and ongoing monitoring while maintaining therapeutic relationships
- Legal and ethical guidelines provide frameworks for confidentiality decisions while ensuring appropriate protection of vulnerable individuals
- Emergency procedures and aftercare planning ensure appropriate crisis response while supporting individual recovery and group stability

- Crisis prevention and resilience building help groups develop skills for managing future challenges while maintaining mutual support and connection

Chapter 16: Integrating Substance Use and Behavioral Addictions

Trauma and addiction dance together in a complex waltz—each partner leading and following in turn, creating patterns that can feel impossible to break. The substances that once numbed unbearable pain become sources of additional shame and suffering, while the trauma that drives addictive behaviors remains unhealed beneath layers of chemical protection. Groups serving individuals with both trauma histories and substance use disorders must address this intertwined relationship with skill, compassion, and realistic expectations about the recovery process.

You cannot treat trauma without addressing the substances that members use to manage it, nor can you treat addiction without healing the wounds that fuel it. This integration requires specialized knowledge, modified protocols, and the wisdom to meet people where they are rather than where you think they should be in their recovery journey.

Trauma-Addiction Interconnections

The relationship between trauma and addiction is so common that many experts consider them a single, integrated condition rather than two separate problems that happen to co-occur. Understanding these connections helps group facilitators develop more effective interventions while reducing the shame and confusion that often surround dual diagnosis presentations.

Self-medication theory explains how individuals use substances to manage trauma symptoms that feel unbearable or overwhelming. Alcohol might quiet hypervigilance and racing thoughts, marijuana could reduce nightmares and insomnia, stimulants may provide energy and focus when depression interferes with functioning, and opioids might numb both physical and emotional pain.

Neurobiological connections between trauma and addiction involve similar brain regions and neurotransmitter systems. Both conditions affect the reward system, stress response, memory processing, and emotional regulation. Chronic substance use can actually worsen trauma symptoms by interfering with natural recovery processes while creating additional neurobiological dysregulation.

Developmental trauma effects on brain development create increased vulnerability to addiction. Individuals who experienced childhood trauma have higher rates of substance use disorders, earlier onset of addiction, more severe addiction patterns, and greater difficulty achieving lasting recovery.

Attachment and addiction share common themes around seeking comfort, avoiding pain, and managing relationships. Substances may become substitute attachment objects that provide reliable comfort when human relationships feel dangerous or unpredictable.

Intergenerational patterns often emerge as trauma and addiction are passed down through families via genetics, modeling, and continued trauma exposure. Family systems may normalize heavy substance use while maintaining trauma-perpetuating dynamics.

Cultural factors influence both trauma exposure and addiction patterns, including how different communities understand and respond to mental health and substance use problems. Some cultures may stigmatize mental health treatment while accepting heavy drinking, creating barriers to integrated treatment.

Robert's trauma and addiction story illustrates these complex interconnections. His combat trauma created severe insomnia, hypervigilance, and emotional numbing that interfered with his relationships and job performance. He began drinking heavily to quiet his racing thoughts and fall asleep, initially finding relief from alcohol's sedating effects.

Over time, Robert's drinking escalated as his tolerance increased and his trauma symptoms worsened. The alcohol that once provided relief began creating additional problems—blackouts that triggered shame

and fear, job performance issues that threatened his security, and relationship conflicts that increased his isolation and distress.

His addiction patterns reflected his military training in several ways: he approached drinking with the same all-or-nothing intensity he brought to other challenges, he used alcohol to maintain emotional control and avoid vulnerability, and he tried to handle his drinking problems through willpower and self-discipline rather than seeking help.

Modified Protocols for Dual Diagnosis Clients

Standard trauma group protocols require significant modifications when working with individuals who have active or recent substance use disorders. These modifications must address the complex interactions between trauma symptoms and substance use while maintaining safety and therapeutic progress for all group members.

Assessment modifications include detailed substance use histories, current use patterns, withdrawal risks, medication interactions, and how substances affect trauma symptoms and therapy participation. This assessment should be ongoing rather than limited to intake, as substance use patterns may change throughout treatment.

Safety considerations become more complex when substances are involved, including increased suicide risk, impaired judgment affecting safety planning, potential for withdrawal symptoms during sessions, and interactions between substances and trauma-related medications.

Group composition decisions require careful thought about mixing individuals with different substances, use patterns, and recovery stages. Some groups work well with mixed populations while others benefit from more homogeneous composition based on primary substance, severity of use, or stage of recovery.

Session modifications might include shorter sessions for individuals with attention problems related to substance use, more frequent check-ins about current use and safety, modified trauma processing techniques that account for potential cognitive impairment, and increased focus on practical coping skills.

Confidentiality complications arise when substance use creates safety concerns or when group members are in treatment programs with different confidentiality requirements. Clear agreements about what information can be shared between programs help protect privacy while ensuring coordination of care.

Homework adaptations recognize that substances may impair memory, motivation, and follow-through on between-session assignments. Modifications might include written reminders, simpler tasks, buddy systems for accountability, and flexible expectations about completion.

Maria's dual diagnosis presentation required significant protocol modifications due to her history of prescription drug misuse following medical procedures for injuries sustained during domestic violence. Her use of prescription pain medications had escalated beyond medical necessity, creating tolerance, withdrawal symptoms, and doctor-shopping behaviors.

The group modifications included more frequent safety check-ins due to her increased suicide risk during withdrawal periods, education about how opioids affect trauma processing and emotional regulation, coordination with her addiction treatment providers, and modified trauma processing techniques that accounted for her cognitive effects from recent substance use.

The group also addressed Maria's shame about her prescription drug problems, which felt different from illegal drug use but created similar patterns of secrecy, denial, and progressive loss of control. The group helped normalize her experience while supporting her recovery efforts.

Harm Reduction vs. Abstinence Approaches

The choice between harm reduction and abstinence-based approaches for trauma groups involving substance use creates ongoing debate among clinicians and affects everything from group composition to intervention strategies. Understanding both approaches helps facilitators make informed decisions based on group member needs and program requirements.

Abstinence-based approaches require complete cessation of alcohol and drug use as a prerequisite for trauma group participation. These approaches argue that substances interfere with trauma processing, emotional regulation development, and authentic relationship building necessary for recovery.

Harm reduction philosophy focuses on reducing negative consequences from substance use rather than requiring complete abstinence. This approach recognizes that many individuals may not be ready or able to achieve abstinence but can still benefit from trauma treatment while working toward reduced use.

Evidence considerations suggest that both approaches can be effective depending on individual circumstances, severity of addiction, stage of change, and availability of support resources. Some individuals require abstinence for any meaningful progress while others make significant trauma recovery progress while continuing modified substance use.

Practical implications of approach choice affect group policies, member selection, crisis management, and relationship with addiction treatment providers. Abstinence-based groups typically require sobriety verification while harm reduction groups focus on honest reporting and safety planning.

Flexibility benefits may come from individualized approaches that recognize different members may need different levels of substance use restriction based on their specific circumstances, substances used, and recovery goals.

Integration challenges arise when group members have different philosophies about substance use or when facilitators must work with both approaches simultaneously within the same program or organization.

Jennifer's situation illustrates the complexity of approach decisions. She had been sober from alcohol for eight months when she joined the trauma group but continued using marijuana occasionally for sleep and anxiety management. Her individual therapist supported this limited use while her AA sponsor disapproved of any substance use.

The trauma group adopted a harm reduction approach for Jennifer, focusing on honest communication about her marijuana use, safety planning around triggers that might lead to alcohol use, and developing non-substance coping strategies while not requiring complete cessation of marijuana use.

This flexible approach allowed Jennifer to participate authentically in trauma treatment while working toward her ultimate goal of complete sobriety. The group supported her recovery efforts without shaming her current use patterns, and she eventually achieved comfortable sobriety from all substances.

Process Addictions in Technology, Sex, and Gambling

Behavioral addictions create similar patterns of compulsive use, negative consequences, and interference with trauma recovery as substance addictions. These process addictions may be less visible than chemical dependencies but can be equally destructive to relationships, functioning, and healing progress.

Technology addiction includes compulsive internet use, social media addiction, gaming addiction, and smartphone dependency. These behaviors may serve similar functions as substances—numbing difficult emotions, avoiding trauma-related thoughts, escaping from current life problems, or seeking stimulation and reward.

Sexual addiction involves compulsive sexual behaviors including pornography use, compulsive masturbation, risky sexual encounters, or multiple affairs. For trauma survivors, sexual addiction may represent attempts to reclaim power and control, seek connection and validation, or recreate trauma dynamics in controllable ways.

Gambling addiction creates cycles of excitement, risk-taking, winning, and losing that can become consuming. For trauma survivors, gambling may provide escape from trauma-related emotions, opportunities for excitement and stimulation, or attempts to solve financial problems created by trauma's impact on functioning.

Shopping and spending addictions involve compulsive purchasing, accumulating debt, and using material acquisitions to manage emotions. These behaviors may represent attempts to fill emotional voids, seek comfort through acquisition, or maintain appearance and status when self-worth feels damaged.

Work addiction includes compulsive overworking, inability to relax or take time off, and using professional achievement to avoid dealing with trauma-related emotions or relationships. Work addiction may be socially acceptable while serving similar avoidance functions as other addictive behaviors.

Assessment challenges for process addictions include cultural normalization of many behaviors, lack of clear diagnostic criteria, and difficulty distinguishing between healthy engagement and addictive patterns.

David's technology addiction became apparent during trauma group when he struggled to put his phone away during sessions, frequently checked social media between group activities, and reported spending 8-10 hours daily on various online activities including gaming, social media, and news consumption.

His technology use served multiple trauma-related functions: online gaming provided escape from intrusive memories and hypervigilance, social media offered superficial connection without vulnerability risks, and constant information consumption kept his mind busy to avoid processing difficult emotions.

The group work addressed his technology addiction as part of his trauma recovery, helping him recognize how excessive online activity interfered with emotional processing, relationship development, and present-moment awareness necessary for healing.

Group Boundaries Around Substance Use

Clear, consistently enforced boundaries around substance use help maintain group safety while providing structure that supports recovery for all members. These boundaries must balance harm reduction principles with safety requirements while addressing the reality that lapses and relapses are common during recovery.

Use reporting requirements establish expectations for honest communication about current substance use, including alcohol, illegal drugs, prescription medications used non-medically, and behavioral addictions. Clear agreements about reporting create safety while reducing shame and secrecy.

Intoxication policies address what happens when group members attend sessions under the influence of substances. Most groups require members to leave if obviously intoxicated, both for safety reasons and because impairment interferes with therapeutic engagement and may trigger other members.

Relapse protocols provide structured responses to substance use episodes that focus on learning and recovery rather than punishment or exclusion. These protocols typically include individual assessment, safety planning, possible temporary group suspension, and clear pathways for returning to group participation.

Sharing guidelines help members discuss substance use experiences appropriately without glorifying use, providing detailed descriptions that might trigger others, or dominating group time with addiction-focused content at the expense of trauma work.

Cross-addiction awareness recognizes that individuals may substitute one addictive behavior for another, requiring attention to various process addictions and behavioral patterns that serve similar functions as primary substances.

Recovery celebration includes acknowledging milestones and progress while being sensitive to members at different recovery stages and avoiding approaches that might trigger competitive dynamics or shame for those struggling with lapses.

Lisa's relapse during group treatment required implementation of established protocols while maintaining her connection to group support. After six months of sobriety, she had several drinking episodes during a particularly difficult period of trauma processing, leading to shame and consideration of dropping out of group.

The group's response followed established protocols: individual assessment of safety and motivation, temporary group suspension while Lisa accessed additional support, development of enhanced safety and recovery planning, and clear agreements about returning to group participation.

The supportive, non-punitive response from both facilitators and group members helped Lisa recommit to her recovery while learning from her relapse experience. She returned to group after two weeks with stronger recovery supports and continued making progress in both addiction recovery and trauma healing.

Medication Considerations and Interactions

Individuals with dual diagnoses often take medications for both trauma-related symptoms and addiction recovery, creating complex medication interactions and considerations that affect group participation and trauma processing work.

Psychiatric medications for trauma symptoms may include antidepressants, mood stabilizers, antipsychotics, or anti-anxiety medications that can affect emotional processing, memory formation, and group participation. Understanding medication effects helps facilitators adjust expectations and interventions appropriately.

Addiction treatment medications such as methadone, buprenorphine, naltrexone, or disulfiram create additional considerations for trauma group work. These medications may affect emotional range, physical comfort, and cognitive functioning in ways that influence therapy participation.

Medication interactions between psychiatric and addiction treatment medications require careful monitoring and coordination between prescribing providers. Changes in one medication may affect the other, requiring adjustments in therapy approaches or group participation.

Withdrawal management may be necessary when individuals are discontinuing substances or changing medications, creating temporary periods of increased vulnerability, emotional instability, or physical discomfort that affect group participation.

Side effect management helps members cope with medication side effects that might interfere with group participation or trauma processing. Common side effects include sedation, cognitive dulling, emotional blunting, or physical symptoms that affect concentration and engagement.

Compliance support recognizes that medication adherence can be challenging for individuals with trauma histories who may have difficulty trusting medical providers or may use medication non-compliance as a form of self-harm or control.

Michael's medication regimen included an antidepressant for trauma-related depression, a mood stabilizer for emotional dysregulation, and naltrexone for alcohol cravings. The interactions between these medications created side effects including cognitive dulling and emotional blunting that affected his group participation.

Working with his psychiatrist, the group facilitator helped advocate for medication adjustments that reduced side effects while maintaining therapeutic benefits. This collaboration improved Michael's ability to engage in trauma processing while maintaining his alcohol recovery.

The group also provided support for Michael's medication adherence challenges, which stemmed partly from his desire to feel emotions fully during trauma processing and partly from his fear of becoming dependent on psychiatric medications as he had been on alcohol.

Integrated Treatment Planning

Effective treatment for individuals with dual diagnoses requires coordination between trauma therapy, addiction treatment, psychiatric care, and other support services. This integration ensures that different treatment approaches complement rather than conflict with each other.

Treatment sequencing decisions involve determining how to balance trauma work with addiction recovery, recognizing that both issues need attention but may require different emphasis at different times. Some individuals need addiction stabilization before trauma work while others can work on both simultaneously.

Provider coordination ensures communication between trauma therapists, addiction counselors, psychiatrists, and other treatment providers. Regular communication helps prevent conflicting approaches while ensuring comprehensive care that addresses all aspects of dual diagnosis presentations.

Goal alignment helps ensure that different treatment providers are working toward compatible goals using consistent approaches. Conflicting treatment philosophies or goals can confuse clients and interfere with progress in all areas.

Crisis planning becomes more complex with dual diagnoses, requiring coordination between trauma crisis resources and addiction crisis services. Clear protocols help ensure appropriate response regardless of which issue precipitates crisis.

Recovery milestones recognition acknowledges progress in both trauma recovery and addiction recovery while understanding that these processes may not proceed at the same pace or in linear fashion.

Sarah's integrated treatment plan included trauma group therapy, individual addiction counseling, psychiatric medication management, and participation in a women's recovery support group. Coordination between providers ensured that her trauma work supported her addiction recovery while her sobriety work enhanced her capacity for trauma processing.

The integrated approach recognized that Sarah's drinking had served important functions in managing trauma symptoms, requiring development of alternative coping strategies before she could maintain comfortable sobriety. Her trauma healing also reduced the emotional pain that had driven her substance use.

Regular communication between providers helped adjust treatment approaches based on Sarah's progress in different areas while ensuring consistent support for both her trauma recovery and addiction recovery goals.

Resilience and Recovery Integration

The ultimate goal of dual diagnosis treatment involves helping individuals develop integrated recovery that addresses both trauma healing and addiction recovery as interconnected processes rather than separate problems requiring separate solutions.

Dual recovery identity involves developing understanding of oneself as someone recovering from both trauma and addiction, recognizing how these experiences interact while building identity around recovery and growth rather than pathology and problems.

Integrated coping strategies provide tools that address both trauma symptoms and substance use triggers simultaneously. These might include mindfulness practices, emotional regulation skills, social support utilization, and meaning-making activities that serve both recovery goals.

Relapse prevention for dual diagnosis requires understanding how trauma symptoms can trigger substance use and how substance use can worsen trauma symptoms. Effective prevention addresses both aspects of the relapse cycle while building resilience in both areas.

Support system development involves building relationships with people who understand and support both trauma recovery and addiction recovery. This might include other group members, recovery community participants, family members, and friends who support integrated recovery.

Purpose and meaning often emerge as individuals develop understanding of how their dual recovery journey can serve broader purposes including helping others, contributing to family healing, or making positive community contributions.

Robert's integrated recovery involved understanding his combat trauma and alcohol addiction as interconnected responses to overwhelming experiences rather than separate character defects or diseases. This understanding reduced his shame while building motivation for addressing both issues simultaneously.

His recovery work included developing coping strategies that addressed both hypervigilance and alcohol cravings, building relationships with other veterans in recovery who understood both experiences, and finding purpose through mentoring other veterans beginning their recovery journeys.

The integration of his trauma healing and addiction recovery created a stronger, more sustainable recovery than addressing either issue in isolation would have achieved.

A Path Forward

Working with dual diagnosis presentations in trauma groups requires specialized knowledge, modified protocols, and integration of multiple treatment approaches. The complexity can feel overwhelming, but the potential for healing is profound when both trauma and addiction are addressed with skill and compassion.

The key lies in understanding trauma and addiction as interconnected conditions that must be treated together rather than sequentially or separately. This integration requires flexibility, patience, and realistic expectations about the recovery process while maintaining hope for lasting healing and growth.

Group treatment offers unique advantages for dual diagnosis work, providing peer support from others who understand both experiences while building recovery community and skills that support long-term success in both areas.

Core Implementation Strategies

- Trauma-addiction interconnections require integrated treatment approaches that address both issues simultaneously rather than separately or sequentially
- Modified protocols for dual diagnosis clients must account for complex interactions between substances and trauma symptoms while maintaining group safety
- Harm reduction versus abstinence decisions should be based on individual needs and circumstances rather than rigid program requirements
- Process addictions require the same attention and treatment approaches as substance addictions while recognizing their trauma-related functions
- Clear group boundaries around substance use maintain safety while supporting recovery through non-punitive, learning-focused approaches
- Integrated treatment planning coordinates multiple providers and approaches while ensuring consistent, comprehensive care for complex presentations

Chapter 17: Specialized Populations and Adaptations

Not all trauma is created equal, and neither are the people who survive it. A combat veteran's moral injury differs profoundly from a refugee's torture survival, just as a first responder's occupational trauma creates different challenges than a healthcare worker's vicarious trauma exposure. Understanding these distinctions matters enormously—not because some traumas are worse than others, but because different populations require different approaches, different understanding, and different kinds of healing environments to recover.

Generic trauma treatment often falls short when applied to specialized populations whose trauma experiences are shaped by unique occupational demands, cultural contexts, or identity factors. Effective group treatment requires adaptation of standard approaches to honor these differences while building on the strengths and resources that different communities bring to the healing process.

First Responders and Occupational Trauma

First responders—police officers, firefighters, paramedics, emergency medical technicians—enter their careers expecting to witness human suffering, but nothing truly prepares them for the accumulated weight of repeated trauma exposure combined with organizational pressures that often discourage seeking help.

Occupational culture considerations profoundly shape how first responders experience and respond to trauma. These cultures typically value stoicism, self-reliance, and emotional control while viewing help-seeking as potential weakness or professional liability. Understanding these cultural factors becomes essential for engaging first responders in meaningful treatment.

Repeated exposure effects create unique trauma presentations where individuals may not identify single traumatic events but instead struggle with the cumulative impact of constant exposure to human suffering, death, and violence. This chronic exposure can lead to emotional numbing, cynicism, and gradual erosion of empathy and connection.

Critical incident stress involves specific traumatic events that exceed normal occupational stressors—mass casualty incidents, line-of-duty deaths, incidents involving children, or situations where the responder knew the victim personally. These critical incidents often trigger acute stress responses that require immediate and specialized intervention.

Moral injury components emerge when first responders witness suffering they cannot prevent, make decisions that conflict with their values under extreme pressure, or experience betrayal by their organizations or colleagues. This moral dimension adds complexity to trauma treatment beyond standard PTSD approaches.

Organizational factors significantly impact both trauma development and recovery, including shift work that disrupts sleep and relationships, bureaucratic constraints that interfere with effective response, lack of organizational support for mental health treatment, and punitive responses to seeking help.

Identity integration challenges arise as first responders must reconcile their professional identity as helpers and protectors with their human vulnerability to trauma and emotional pain. This integration often requires addressing beliefs about strength, vulnerability, and professional competence.

Captain Martinez, a 15-year veteran of the fire department, joined a first responder trauma group after struggling with increasing anxiety, insomnia, and emotional distance from his family. His trauma history included numerous structure fires, vehicle accidents, and medical emergencies, but he particularly struggled with a house fire where he couldn't save two children despite heroic efforts.

The specialized group approach honored his professional identity while addressing the ways his occupational culture had taught him to suppress emotional responses that were now creating problems in his personal life. The group included other firefighters, police officers, and paramedics who understood the unique pressures of first responder work.

Treatment adaptations included scheduling sessions during off-duty hours, using terminology familiar to first responders, addressing practical concerns about confidentiality and career impact, and building on the natural camaraderie and mutual support that exists within first responder communities.

Healthcare Workers and Vicarious Trauma

Healthcare workers face unique trauma challenges through constant exposure to human suffering, death, and ethical dilemmas while maintaining professional responsibilities for patient care. The COVID-19 pandemic intensified these challenges while highlighting the mental health needs of healthcare professionals.

Vicarious trauma development occurs through repeated exposure to patient trauma stories, witnessing patient suffering and death, and absorbing the emotional pain of patients and families. This secondary trauma exposure can create symptoms similar to direct trauma while being less recognized and validated.

Compassion fatigue represents the physical, mental, and emotional exhaustion that results from caring for patients in significant emotional distress. This fatigue can lead to decreased empathy, increased cynicism, and reduced professional satisfaction that affects both personal wellbeing and patient care quality.

Moral distress arises when healthcare workers know the right action to take but are prevented from taking it due to institutional constraints, resource limitations, or system failures. This distress creates internal conflict between professional values and practical realities that can be deeply traumatizing.

Professional identity conflicts emerge when healthcare workers struggle to reconcile their role as healers with their human limitations and emotional needs. The expectation to remain strong and composed while repeatedly witnessing trauma can create internal pressure that interferes with natural processing and healing.

Systemic pressures include heavy caseloads, documentation requirements, insurance limitations, and organizational demands that leave little time for self-care or emotional processing. These systemic factors can perpetuate trauma while making it difficult to access or engage in treatment.

Boundary challenges arise as healthcare workers struggle to maintain appropriate emotional boundaries with patients while providing compassionate care. Both over-involvement and emotional detachment can create problems, requiring careful balance between professional effectiveness and personal protection.

Dr. Sarah Kim, an emergency room physician, sought group treatment after experiencing panic attacks, intrusive memories of patient deaths, and increasing alcohol use to manage work-related stress. Her trauma exposure included treating victims of violence, conducting death notifications, and making life-or-death decisions under pressure.

The healthcare worker trauma group provided understanding of the unique challenges facing medical professionals while addressing the ways medical training had taught participants to intellectualize rather than process emotional responses to traumatic patient encounters.

Group adaptations included flexible scheduling to accommodate unpredictable healthcare schedules, addressing confidentiality concerns related to professional licensing, and developing coping strategies that could be used during work shifts without interfering with patient care responsibilities.

Combat Veterans and Moral Injury

Military trauma extends beyond traditional PTSD to include moral injury—the damage that occurs when service members perpetrate, witness, or fail to prevent acts that violate their moral beliefs and expectations. This moral dimension requires specialized treatment approaches that address both trauma symptoms and spiritual/ethical wounds.

Combat exposure variations include direct combat with enemy forces, witnessing injury or death of fellow service members, being injured in combat, handling remains of dead bodies, and experiencing near-death situations. Each type of exposure creates different trauma presentations requiring individualized treatment approaches.

Moral injury dimensions involve perpetration (actions taken that violate moral beliefs), betrayal (being let down by trusted others in high-stakes situations), and witnessing (observing acts that violate moral expectations). These moral injuries often create more persistent distress than traditional trauma symptoms.

Military culture factors emphasize honor, courage, loyalty, and sacrifice while discouraging emotional vulnerability or help-seeking. These cultural values can both support resilience and create barriers to treatment engagement and emotional processing.

Transition challenges from military to civilian life involve losing structured environment, clear mission and purpose, close-knit unit relationships, and respect for military service. These losses can compound trauma symptoms while making civilian life feel meaningless or unsatisfying.

Identity reconstruction becomes necessary as veterans integrate their military experiences with civilian life while maintaining positive aspects of military identity. This reconstruction involves grieving losses while building new sources of meaning and purpose.

Spiritual considerations often emerge as veterans struggle with questions about God, justice, meaning, and their place in the world after experiencing extreme violence and moral complexity.

Traditional religious frameworks may feel inadequate for processing combat experiences.

Sergeant First Class Johnson joined a combat veteran trauma group after struggling with nightmares, survivor guilt, and rage following multiple deployments to Afghanistan. His moral injury centered on a convoy incident where his decisions led to civilian casualties, creating intense guilt and self-blame that persisted despite understanding the impossible circumstances he faced.

The veteran-focused group provided understanding of military culture and combat experiences while addressing the spiritual and moral dimensions of his trauma. Other group members shared similar experiences of making impossible decisions under combat conditions, helping normalize his responses while supporting his healing process.

Treatment adaptations included using military terminology and concepts, addressing transition challenges from military to civilian life, involving family members who struggled to understand combat trauma, and connecting him with veteran service organizations for ongoing support.

Refugees and Torture Survivors

Refugees and torture survivors face complex trauma that often includes pre-migration persecution, torture, and violence; dangerous migration journeys; and post-migration challenges including cultural adjustment, language barriers, and ongoing discrimination or deportation fears.

Pre-migration trauma may include war exposure, political persecution, ethnic cleansing, torture, sexual violence, and witnessing atrocities. These experiences often occur over extended periods and may involve betrayal by trusted community members or government authorities.

Migration trauma includes dangerous border crossings, family separation, detention experiences, and uncertainty about destination and safety. The migration process itself can be traumatizing while individuals are already vulnerable from pre-migration experiences.

Post-migration stressors include cultural adjustment challenges, language barriers, employment difficulties, discrimination, poverty, and ongoing fears about deportation or family safety. These stressors can perpetuate trauma symptoms while interfering with recovery and integration.

Torture survivor needs require specialized understanding of both physical and psychological torture effects, including complex PTSD presentations, dissociation, somatization, and difficulty trusting authority figures including therapists.

Cultural considerations involve understanding diverse cultural backgrounds, religious beliefs, and explanatory models for mental health and healing. Treatment must be adapted to honor cultural values while providing effective trauma intervention.

Legal and advocacy needs often require coordination with immigration attorneys, human rights organizations, and social service agencies that provide practical assistance with asylum claims, family reunification, and basic survival needs.

Fatima, a refugee from Syria, joined a specialized refugee trauma group after experiencing depression, anxiety, and intrusive memories related to war experiences, torture during detention, and dangerous journey to the United States. Her trauma was compounded by ongoing concerns about family members still in Syria and uncertainty about her asylum claim.

The refugee-focused group included participants from various countries who shared experiences of persecution, displacement, and cultural adjustment. The group provided validation for experiences that many Americans could not understand while addressing practical concerns about safety and legal status.

Treatment adaptations included using interpreters when needed, incorporating cultural healing practices, coordinating with legal advocates working on asylum claims, and addressing practical needs for housing, employment, and healthcare that affected mental health recovery.

LGBTQ+ Individuals and Minority Stress

LGBTQ+ individuals often experience unique forms of trauma related to their sexual orientation or gender identity, including family rejection, discrimination, violence, and internalized shame. These experiences require specialized treatment approaches that address both direct trauma and minority stress effects.

Minority stress factors include distal stressors (external experiences of discrimination and violence) and proximal stressors (internal processes like internalized homophobia and identity concealment). These stressors create chronic stress that can compound other trauma experiences.

Identity development challenges involve navigating sexual orientation or gender identity development in hostile or non-affirming environments. This development may be complicated by trauma experiences that interfere with healthy identity formation and self-acceptance.

Family rejection trauma can be particularly devastating as it involves rejection by those expected to provide love and support. This rejection may include emotional, physical, or financial cutoff that creates ongoing trauma and instability.

Discrimination and violence based on LGBTQ+ identity can range from microaggressions and subtle discrimination to physical violence and hate crimes. These experiences often involve unpredictability and targeting of core identity aspects.

Internalized oppression involves absorbing negative societal messages about LGBTQ+ identities, leading to self-hatred, shame, and internal conflict about identity and relationships. This internalized oppression can be more damaging than external discrimination.

Institutional discrimination includes barriers to healthcare, employment, housing, and other services that create ongoing stress while limiting access to resources needed for trauma recovery.

Alex, a transgender man, joined an LGBTQ+ trauma group after experiencing depression and anxiety related to family rejection following his transition, workplace discrimination, and physical assault motivated by transphobia. His trauma was compounded by internalized shame about his gender identity and fears about safety in public spaces.

The LGBTQ+-affirming group provided validation for experiences that heterosexual, cisgender therapists might not fully understand while addressing both external trauma experiences and internal struggles with identity acceptance and minority stress.

Treatment adaptations included using chosen names and pronouns, addressing internalized oppression and shame, developing safety planning for discrimination and violence, and building positive LGBTQ+ identity and community connections.

Cultural Adaptation Principles

Effective adaptation of trauma treatment for specialized populations requires understanding unique cultural factors, trauma presentations, and healing traditions while maintaining core elements of effective trauma intervention.

Cultural competence development involves ongoing education about different populations, examination of personal biases and assumptions, and development of skills for working across cultural differences. This competence must be genuine rather than superficial tokenism.

Language adaptation may require using interpreters, learning key terms in other languages, or adapting concepts to fit different cultural frameworks. Simple translation is often insufficient; concepts may need fundamental reframing to be meaningful across cultures.

Healing tradition integration involves learning about and incorporating traditional healing practices from different cultures while respecting their integrity and meaning. This integration should be done with community input rather than therapist assumptions about what might be helpful.

Community involvement helps ensure that treatment approaches are acceptable and effective within specific cultural contexts. Community leaders, cultural consultants, and peer support from similar backgrounds can enhance treatment effectiveness.

Advocacy and social justice components may be necessary when trauma is related to ongoing oppression or discrimination. Individual healing may require addressing systemic factors that continue creating trauma and limiting recovery.

Outcome measurement must be adapted to be culturally relevant and meaningful within different populations. Standard measures may not capture important aspects of healing or may be biased toward dominant cultural perspectives.

The refugee trauma program developed cultural adaptations including partnerships with ethnic community organizations, training for therapists in refugee experiences and cultural factors, integration of traditional healing practices where appropriate, and advocacy for policy changes affecting refugee mental health access.

These adaptations improved both treatment engagement and outcomes while building community trust and support for mental health services. The program became a model for culturally responsive trauma treatment in the region.

Building Specialized Expertise

Developing expertise in specialized population trauma treatment requires ongoing education, consultation, and supervision while building relationships with communities and organizations serving specific populations.

Training requirements include formal education about specific populations, supervised experience with specialized trauma presentations, and ongoing consultation with experts in cultural adaptation and specialized trauma treatment.

Community relationships help therapists understand population needs, cultural factors, and available resources while building trust and credibility within specific communities. These relationships should be genuine partnerships rather than one-way consultation.

Organizational support provides backing for specialized program development, cultural adaptation efforts, and community outreach activities. Organizations must commit resources and support rather than expecting individual therapists to develop expertise without backing.

Outcome tracking helps demonstrate effectiveness of specialized approaches while identifying areas needing improvement or adaptation. This tracking should include both clinical outcomes and community satisfaction measures.

Program sustainability requires ongoing funding, staff training, and community support to maintain specialized services over time. Specialized programs often require different funding models and sustainability strategies than general trauma services.

The first responder trauma program developed expertise through partnerships with fire departments, police agencies, and EMS services; specialized training for therapists in occupational trauma and first responder culture; and ongoing consultation with active and retired first responders who provided cultural guidance and credibility within these communities.

Honoring Diversity in Healing

Specialized population trauma treatment represents more than clinical adaptation—it's recognition that healing happens within cultural contexts and that effective treatment must honor the diversity of human experience while building on community strengths and wisdom.

The goal is not to create completely separate treatment approaches but to adapt evidence-based interventions in ways that make them accessible, acceptable, and effective across different populations while maintaining core elements that promote healing and recovery.

This work requires humility, ongoing learning, and genuine respect for different cultures and communities while building bridges between professional mental health approaches and traditional healing wisdom that communities have developed over generations.

Specialized Treatment Foundations

- First responder trauma treatment must address occupational culture factors while honoring professional identity and building on natural peer support systems
- Healthcare worker programs require understanding of vicarious trauma, moral distress, and professional identity conflicts unique to medical settings
- Combat veteran services must address moral injury dimensions while supporting military identity integration and civilian transition challenges
- Refugee and torture survivor treatment requires cultural adaptation, interpreter services, and coordination with legal and advocacy resources
- LGBTQ+ specialized approaches must address minority stress, identity development challenges, and internalized oppression in affirming environments
- Cultural adaptation principles guide modification of standard treatments while maintaining effectiveness and honoring diverse healing traditions

Chapter 18: Assessment Tools and Outcome Measurement

Numbers tell stories, but not always the ones we expect. A perfectly completed questionnaire might hide behind-the-scenes chaos, while someone who struggles with formal measures could be making profound changes that standardized instruments fail to capture. Assessment in trauma group work requires balancing scientific rigor with clinical intuition, using measurement tools that inform rather than constrain the therapeutic process.

The art lies in choosing assessments that capture meaningful change while avoiding the trap of reducing complex human healing to simple scores. Effective measurement serves both clinical needs—helping guide treatment decisions and track progress—and research requirements that demonstrate treatment effectiveness and support program sustainability.

Pre-treatment Assessment Battery

A thorough pre-treatment assessment provides the foundation for all subsequent treatment planning, outcome measurement, and program evaluation. This battery must be extensive enough to capture the complexity of trauma presentations while remaining feasible for clients who may be overwhelmed, suspicious of formal procedures, or limited by cognitive or educational factors.

Trauma history assessment forms the cornerstone of pre-treatment evaluation, requiring instruments that capture both objective trauma exposure and subjective trauma impact. This assessment should include childhood trauma, adult trauma, multiple trauma exposure, and cultural/historical trauma experiences that shape individual presentations.

Symptom severity measures provide baseline data about current functioning across multiple domains including PTSD symptoms, depression, anxiety, dissociation, and other trauma-related presentations. These measures should be sensitive to change while providing normative data for comparison purposes.

Functional impairment assessment examines how trauma symptoms affect daily life including work performance, relationship functioning, parenting capacity, self-care abilities, and social engagement. This functional focus often provides more meaningful information than symptom severity alone.

Strengths and resources identification balances deficit-focused assessment with recognition of individual and cultural resources that support healing. This might include coping strategies, social support, spiritual resources, cultural connections, and previous successful change experiences.

Readiness for group treatment evaluation includes factors like motivation for change, ability to tolerate group settings, capacity for emotional regulation, and realistic expectations about group therapy process and outcomes.

Risk assessment covers suicide risk, self-harm behaviors, substance abuse, violence potential, and other safety concerns that might affect group participation or require specialized intervention approaches.

Jennifer's pre-treatment assessment revealed complex trauma presentations including childhood sexual abuse, domestic violence, and recent sexual assault. Her symptom measures showed severe PTSD, moderate depression, and significant dissociation with high functional impairment across work, relationships, and self-care domains.

However, her assessment also revealed significant strengths including strong spiritual beliefs, supportive relationship with her sister, artistic abilities that provided emotional expression, and previous therapy experience that included some symptom improvement. Her motivation for group treatment was high, and she demonstrated capacity for self-reflection and emotional expression.

The comprehensive assessment guided treatment planning by identifying targets for intervention, potential triggers to monitor, resources to build upon, and modifications needed to support her successful group participation.

Session-by-session Monitoring Tools

Regular monitoring throughout treatment provides essential feedback about progress, emerging issues, and need for treatment modifications. These tools must be brief enough for routine use while sensitive enough to detect meaningful change and potential deterioration.

Weekly symptom tracking involves brief measures that can be completed before each session, providing information about current symptom levels, recent stressors, and response to previous session content. These measures help therapists adjust session focus based on current needs.

Session impact assessment measures immediate responses to group sessions including emotional reactions, perceived helpfulness, triggering content, and overall session satisfaction. This feedback helps facilitators modify approaches and content based on group response.

Between-session functioning includes measures of daily functioning, coping strategy use, substance use patterns, and application of skills learned in group sessions. This information helps bridge therapy and daily life application.

Goal progress tracking provides regular assessment of movement toward individual treatment goals using personally meaningful metrics rather than only standardized measures. This tracking maintains focus on individual priorities and values.

Group dynamics assessment measures members' perceptions of group climate, cohesion, safety, and therapeutic factors. This information helps facilitators address group process issues that might interfere with individual progress.

Crisis and safety monitoring includes regular assessment of suicide risk, self-harm behaviors, substance use escalation, and other safety concerns that require immediate attention and intervention.

Maria's weekly monitoring revealed that her PTSD symptoms typically spiked following sessions that included trauma processing but then decreased to below baseline levels within a few days. This pattern helped the facilitator understand that temporary symptom increases actually indicated therapeutic progress rather than treatment failure.

Her session impact assessments showed that she found imagery rescripting particularly helpful while chair work initially felt threatening and overwhelming. This feedback guided modifications to her individual treatment approach within the group setting.

The monitoring also revealed that Maria was applying grounding techniques successfully at home but struggling to use interpersonal skills with her husband, leading to additional focus on relationship applications during group sessions.

Group Climate and Cohesion Measures

Group process factors significantly influence individual outcomes, making measurement of group dynamics essential for both clinical and research purposes. These measures help identify when group interventions are needed while tracking the development of therapeutic group conditions.

Group cohesion assessment measures the degree to which group members feel connected to each other and committed to group goals. High cohesion generally predicts better individual outcomes while low cohesion may indicate need for group process interventions.

Therapeutic factor identification assesses which group therapeutic factors members experience as most helpful including universality, instillation of hope, interpersonal learning, catharsis, and corrective recapitulation of family dynamics.

Group climate evaluation measures overall group atmosphere including warmth, support, expressiveness, and emotional safety. Positive group climate supports individual risk-taking and therapeutic engagement while negative climate may require intervention.

Conflict and tension tracking identifies interpersonal difficulties, subgroup formation, scapegoating patterns, and other group dynamics that might interfere with therapeutic progress for individual members or the group as whole.

Leadership and participation patterns assess how different members contribute to group functioning including helpful behaviors, disruptive behaviors, and patterns of participation that affect group effectiveness.

Group development stages tracking helps facilitators understand whether groups are progressing through normal developmental stages or becoming stuck in unproductive patterns that require intervention.

Robert's group cohesion scores remained low during the first eight sessions, reflecting his difficulty connecting with other members and trusting the group process. This information guided individual interventions to address his attachment difficulties while helping the group develop patience with his gradual engagement process.

The group's therapeutic factor ratings showed high scores for universality and instillation of hope but lower scores for interpersonal learning, suggesting that members were benefiting from shared experiences but not yet challenging each other's patterns or providing direct feedback.

This information led to facilitator interventions that encouraged more direct interpersonal feedback while maintaining the safety and support that members valued most about their group experience.

211

Trauma Symptom Tracking Instruments

Specialized trauma measures provide detailed information about specific symptom clusters while tracking changes in areas most relevant to trauma recovery. These instruments should be selected based on individual presentations while maintaining consistency for comparison purposes.

PTSD symptom measures assess intrusion symptoms, avoidance behaviors, negative alterations in mood and cognition, and hyperarousal symptoms as defined by current diagnostic criteria. These measures should distinguish between different symptom clusters that may respond differently to treatment.

Complex trauma assessment evaluates emotional dysregulation, negative self-concept, and interpersonal difficulties that characterize complex PTSD presentations. These measures capture trauma effects that extend beyond traditional PTSD symptoms.

Dissociation tracking measures different types of dissociative experiences including depersonalization, derealization, amnesia, and identity confusion. These symptoms often require specialized attention and may affect ability to engage in standard trauma treatments.

Somatic symptom assessment evaluates physical symptoms that may be trauma-related including chronic pain, gastrointestinal problems, sleep disturbances, and other bodily manifestations of trauma that might not be captured by psychological measures alone.

Attachment and relationship measures assess capacity for healthy relationships, trust, intimacy, and interpersonal effectiveness that are often impaired by trauma experiences and represent important treatment targets.

Post-traumatic growth assessment measures positive changes that may result from trauma recovery including appreciation of life, relating to others, personal strength awareness, spiritual development, and new possibilities recognition.

David's trauma symptom tracking revealed that his intrusion symptoms (nightmares, flashbacks) improved more quickly than his avoidance symptoms (social withdrawal, emotional numbing), helping the treatment team understand his specific recovery pattern and adjust interventions accordingly.

His dissociation scores remained elevated even as other symptoms improved, leading to additional focus on grounding techniques and parts integration work. The tracking also revealed that his somatic symptoms (chronic back pain, insomnia) were closely linked to his emotional state and trauma processing work.

The comprehensive tracking helped identify which interventions were most effective for his specific presentation while providing motivation as he could see objective evidence of his recovery progress over time.

Long-term Follow-up Protocols

Long-term outcome assessment provides essential information about treatment durability while identifying factors that support sustained recovery versus risk for symptom return. These protocols must balance research needs with practical limitations of maintaining contact with former group members.

Follow-up timing typically includes assessments at treatment completion, three months post-treatment, six months post-treatment, and one year post-treatment. Some studies extend follow-up to two or more years to assess long-term durability of treatment effects.

Outcome domains should include symptom levels, functional impairment, quality of life, relationship functioning, work performance, and other areas that reflect meaningful life change beyond symptom reduction alone.

Maintenance strategy assessment evaluates what former group members are doing to maintain their recovery progress including continued individual therapy, peer support participation, self-care practices, and skill application in daily life.

Relapse and setback tracking identifies factors that contribute to symptom return or functional deterioration while assessing how individuals cope with inevitable life challenges and stressors.

Service utilization measures use of mental health services, medical services, and other support resources following group treatment completion, providing information about ongoing needs and treatment gaps.

Satisfaction and helpfulness evaluation assesses former members' retrospective perceptions of group treatment including most helpful components, suggested improvements, and likelihood of recommending treatment to others.

Lisa's six-month follow-up revealed that her trauma symptoms remained significantly improved compared to pre-treatment levels, but she had experienced some increase in depression during a difficult period at work. Her follow-up interview revealed that she was successfully using coping strategies learned in group but had stopped practicing mindfulness exercises regularly.

The follow-up information guided recommendations for booster sessions focusing on depression management and renewed commitment to daily mindfulness practice. Lisa's experience also informed program modifications to include more emphasis on maintenance planning during group treatment.

Her feedback that group members' ongoing contact had been crucial for maintaining progress led to development of formal alumni group opportunities for former participants who wanted continued peer support.

Technology-Enhanced Assessment

Digital tools increasingly support assessment and monitoring processes while providing advantages in data collection, analysis, and participant convenience. However, technology must be implemented thoughtfully to enhance rather than replace human clinical judgment.

Mobile app integration allows for real-time symptom tracking, mood monitoring, and ecological momentary assessment that captures experiences as they occur rather than relying on retrospective reporting. These tools can provide rich data about symptom patterns and trigger identification.

Online survey platforms facilitate administration of assessment batteries while reducing staff time and improving data quality through automatic skip patterns, range checks, and immediate scoring. These platforms must maintain appropriate security and privacy protections.

Wearable device data from fitness trackers, smartwatches, and other devices can provide objective information about sleep patterns, activity levels, heart rate variability, and other physiological markers that may reflect trauma recovery progress.

Video and audio analysis using artificial intelligence tools may eventually provide objective measures of affect, speech patterns, and other indicators of psychological state that complement self-report measures.

Virtual reality assessment environments can provide standardized trigger exposure for assessment purposes while measuring physiological and behavioral responses in controlled, replicable conditions.

Data integration challenges include combining information from multiple sources while maintaining privacy protection and ensuring that technology enhances rather than complicates clinical decision-making processes.

Michael's program piloted smartphone app-based daily monitoring that allowed him to track sleep quality, anxiety levels, substance use urges, and coping strategy use. The data revealed patterns he hadn't

215

noticed including increased anxiety on weekends and better sleep quality following days when he exercised.

The objective data from his fitness tracker showed gradual improvements in sleep efficiency and heart rate variability that correlated with his subjective reports of reduced hypervigilance and better emotional regulation.

However, the technology also created some burden as Michael sometimes felt pressured to complete assessments even when he was busy or distressed, highlighting the need for flexible approaches that support rather than stress participants.

Data-Driven Treatment Decisions

Assessment information becomes valuable only when it's used to guide clinical decisions and improve treatment outcomes. This requires systematic approaches to data review, interpretation, and application that inform rather than replace clinical judgment.

Progress monitoring protocols establish regular review of assessment data with clear decision points about when to modify treatment approaches, when to celebrate progress, and when to consider alternative interventions.

Treatment matching uses assessment information to assign individuals to interventions most likely to be effective for their specific presentations while avoiding one-size-fits-all approaches that may not meet individual needs.

Risk management systems use assessment data to identify individuals at increased risk for deterioration, dropout, or crisis while implementing preventive interventions before problems escalate.

Outcome prediction models may eventually use assessment data to predict which individuals are most likely to benefit from specific interventions while identifying those who may need enhanced or alternative approaches.

Quality improvement processes use aggregate assessment data to identify program strengths and weaknesses while implementing systematic improvements based on participant feedback and outcome data.

Research integration connects clinical assessment data with research efforts that advance understanding of trauma treatment while ensuring that clinical programs benefit from research findings.

Sarah's assessment data revealed that her progress stalled after eight sessions despite initial improvement, leading to treatment modifications including additional individual sessions, medication consultation, and enhanced trauma processing approaches.

The data-driven decision-making helped identify that her plateau coincided with increased work stress and relationship conflicts, leading to interventions that addressed these concurrent issues rather than only focusing on trauma symptoms.

Her positive response to treatment modifications validated the importance of ongoing monitoring and flexible treatment approaches that can be adjusted based on individual progress patterns and changing life circumstances.

Measuring What Matters

Assessment in trauma group work serves healing when it captures meaningful change while avoiding the trap of reducing complex human experiences to numbers and scores. The goal is creating measurement approaches that inform clinical decision-making while honoring the complexity and individuality of trauma recovery.

Effective assessment balances scientific rigor with clinical practicality, using tools that enhance understanding while avoiding burden that interferes with therapeutic relationships or treatment engagement. The best measures provide information that helps individuals understand their own progress while guiding interventions that support continued healing.

The ultimate test of assessment effectiveness lies not in the sophistication of the instruments but in how well the information supports better treatment decisions, improved outcomes, and enhanced understanding of what helps people heal from trauma.

Key Assessment Principles

- Pre-treatment assessment batteries provide essential baseline information while identifying strengths, resources, and treatment targets for individual participants
- Session-by-session monitoring tools offer ongoing feedback about progress, emerging issues, and need for treatment modifications
- Group climate and cohesion measures help identify group process factors that influence individual outcomes and guide group interventions
- Trauma symptom tracking instruments provide detailed information about specific symptom clusters while measuring areas most relevant to recovery
- Long-term follow-up protocols assess treatment durability while identifying factors that support sustained recovery versus relapse risk
- Technology-enhanced assessment can improve data quality and convenience while requiring thoughtful implementation that enhances rather than burdens treatment

Chapter 19: Technology Integration and Hybrid Delivery

The therapy room has expanded beyond four walls—stretching through fiber optic cables into living rooms, connecting through smartphone screens, and creating healing spaces that exist somewhere between physical and digital reality. Technology integration in trauma group work isn't simply about convenience or pandemic adaptation; it's about fundamentally rethinking how healing relationships form and therapeutic communities develop when geography, mobility, and circumstance no longer limit who can participate.

Yet technology brings both promise and peril to trauma treatment. The same tools that can connect isolated survivors and provide 24-hour support can also trigger symptoms, compromise privacy, and create new forms of disconnection. The challenge lies in harnessing technology's benefits while mitigating its risks, creating therapeutic experiences that honor trauma survivors' needs for safety, connection, and authentic relationship.

Telehealth Group Therapy Best Practices

Online group therapy requires fundamental adaptations of traditional approaches while maintaining the therapeutic factors that make group treatment effective. These adaptations must address technical, clinical, and relational challenges that don't exist in face-to-face settings.

Platform selection involves choosing technology that balances security, functionality, and user-friendliness while meeting healthcare privacy requirements. The platform must support group interactions, breakout rooms, screen sharing, and recording capabilities while maintaining HIPAA compliance and providing reliable service.

Environment optimization helps both facilitators and participants create spaces that support therapeutic engagement while maintaining privacy and minimizing distractions. This includes lighting, camera positioning, background considerations, and noise management strategies.

Technical preparation ensures that all participants have necessary equipment, internet connectivity, and technical skills to participate effectively. This may require providing devices, internet support, or technical training for participants who lack resources or experience.

Engagement strategies adapt traditional group techniques for online delivery while developing new approaches that leverage technology's unique capabilities. This includes using chat functions, virtual backgrounds, breakout rooms, and collaborative tools that enhance rather than distract from therapeutic process.

Crisis management protocols address how to handle psychiatric emergencies when participants may be in remote locations without immediate support available. This requires knowing participants' locations, emergency contacts, and local crisis resources.

Confidentiality considerations become more complex when participants join from home environments where family members, roommates, or others might overhear sessions or when technical issues might compromise privacy.

Sarah joined an online trauma group after struggling to find in-person treatment in her rural area. The telehealth format allowed her to access specialized trauma treatment while managing childcare responsibilities that would have made in-person attendance impossible.

The group facilitator helped Sarah optimize her environment by finding a private space in her home, using headphones to protect confidentiality, and developing strategies for managing interruptions from her children during sessions.

The online format actually reduced Sarah's anxiety about group participation initially, as she felt safer sharing from her own home environment. However, she later found that the physical distance made it harder to feel connected to other group members, requiring additional interventions to build group cohesion.

Digital Tools for Homework and Monitoring

Technology can extend therapeutic work beyond session boundaries while providing tools for skill practice, symptom monitoring, and crisis support. These digital interventions must be carefully integrated with group treatment to enhance rather than replace human connection and professional guidance.

Symptom tracking apps allow participants to monitor their emotional states, trigger exposure, and coping strategy use in real-time while providing data that informs treatment planning and progress assessment. These apps must be user-friendly while protecting sensitive mental health information.

Skill practice platforms provide guided exercises for breathing techniques, mindfulness practices, grounding strategies, and other coping skills learned in group sessions. Interactive elements can make practice more engaging while providing feedback about technique and progress.

Peer support networks facilitated through secure messaging or forum platforms allow group members to maintain connection between sessions while providing mutual support during difficult times. These networks require clear guidelines and monitoring to maintain safety and therapeutic boundaries.

Crisis support tools include 24-hour access to crisis resources, safety planning applications, and emergency contact systems that provide immediate support when professional services aren't immediately available.

Psychoeducation resources delivered through video, podcast, or interactive formats can reinforce learning from group sessions while providing additional information about trauma, recovery, and self-care practices.

Progress visualization tools help participants track their recovery journey through graphs, charts, or other visual representations that make progress concrete and motivating while identifying patterns and trends in symptom improvement.

Michael used a trauma recovery app that allowed him to track his sleep quality, anxiety levels, and use of coping strategies on a daily basis. The app provided gentle reminders to practice breathing exercises and offered guided meditations specifically designed for trauma survivors.

The data from Michael's app revealed patterns he hadn't noticed—his anxiety spiked on Sunday evenings before the work week, and his sleep improved significantly on days when he practiced progressive muscle relaxation. This information helped the group facilitator tailor interventions to his specific patterns.

The app also connected Michael with other group members through a secure messaging feature that allowed them to share encouragement and support between sessions. This peer connection proved especially valuable during a difficult period when Michael was processing combat memories and needed additional support.

Virtual Reality Applications for Exposure Work

Virtual reality technology offers new possibilities for trauma treatment by creating controlled exposure experiences that can be precisely calibrated to individual tolerance levels while maintaining the safety of the therapeutic environment.

Exposure therapy enhancement allows for gradual, systematic exposure to trauma-related triggers in controlled virtual environments that can be adjusted based on individual response and progress. This technology provides consistency and safety that may not be available in real-world exposure exercises.

Environmental recreation can help participants process traumatic experiences by recreating locations or situations relevant to their trauma while maintaining complete control over the experience and immediate access to support and grounding resources.

Skills practice environments provide opportunities to rehearse coping strategies, interpersonal skills, and other therapeutic techniques in realistic but safe virtual settings before applying them in real-world situations.

Immersive relaxation experiences can transport participants to calming environments like peaceful beaches, mountain scenes, or other settings that promote nervous system regulation and emotional healing.

Social skills training platforms allow participants to practice interpersonal interactions, public speaking, or other anxiety-provoking social situations in low-stakes virtual environments before attempting them in person.

Assessment applications can provide standardized trigger exposure for research purposes while measuring physiological responses, emotional reactions, and behavioral changes in controlled, replicable conditions.

Jennifer used virtual reality exposure therapy to address her fear of driving, which had developed after a car accident that triggered memories of childhood sexual abuse. The VR system allowed her to gradually practice driving scenarios while remaining physically safe in the therapist's office.

The virtual environment could be precisely calibrated to her tolerance level—starting with sitting in a parked car, progressing to driving in empty parking lots, and eventually practicing highway driving during rush hour traffic. Her physiological responses were monitored throughout to ensure she remained within her window of tolerance.

The VR exposure work was integrated with her group therapy, where she could process her experiences and receive support from other members who understood trauma-related phobias and avoidance behaviors.

App-Based Interventions and Supplements

Mobile applications can provide powerful supplements to group therapy by offering on-demand access to therapeutic tools, educational resources, and support networks. However, these apps must be carefully selected and integrated to ensure they enhance rather than replace human therapeutic relationships.

Evidence-based app selection involves choosing applications that have research support and clinical validation rather than relying on marketing claims or popular appeal. Apps should complement group therapy goals while providing genuine therapeutic benefit.

Customization capabilities allow apps to be tailored to individual needs, trauma types, and skill levels while providing personalization that makes tools more relevant and engaging for specific users.

Integration strategies connect app use with group therapy content by assigning specific exercises, reviewing app data during sessions, and using technology insights to guide treatment planning and goal setting.

Privacy and security considerations become crucial when recommending apps that collect sensitive mental health information. Participants need clear information about data collection, storage, and sharing practices.

Digital literacy support may be necessary for participants who have limited experience with technology or who need assistance learning to use therapeutic apps effectively.

Outcome tracking helps determine which apps are most helpful for different individuals while identifying features that enhance versus interfere with therapeutic progress.

Lisa used a combination of apps including a mood tracking tool, a guided meditation platform, and a crisis support application that provided immediate access to coping strategies and emergency resources. The apps were integrated with her group therapy through weekly reviews of her tracking data and discussion of which tools she found most helpful.

The mood tracking app revealed that Lisa's emotional states were closely linked to sleep quality and social interactions, leading to group discussions about sleep hygiene and interpersonal skills. The meditation app provided guided practices specifically designed for trauma survivors, which Lisa found more helpful than generic mindfulness apps.

However, Lisa also found that some apps increased her anxiety by focusing too much on monitoring and measurement rather than healing and growth. This experience led to careful selection of apps that matched her personality and recovery style.

Maintaining Therapeutic Alliance Remotely

Building and maintaining therapeutic relationships through digital interfaces requires adaptation of traditional alliance-building techniques while developing new approaches that leverage technology's unique possibilities for connection.

Presence and attunement skills must be adapted for online environments where subtle nonverbal cues may be harder to detect and respond to. Facilitators need enhanced skills in reading online behavior while conveying warmth and understanding through digital media.

Technical competence becomes part of therapeutic competence as facilitators must manage technology smoothly while maintaining focus on therapeutic process. Technical difficulties can disrupt therapeutic relationships if not handled skillfully.

Boundary considerations become more complex when therapy moves into participants' homes through technology. Clear agreements about session boundaries, emergency contact, and appropriate use of technology help maintain professional relationships.

Personal connection strategies may need enhancement in online environments where natural rapport-building may be more challenging. This might include longer check-in periods, smaller group sizes, or additional individual contact.

Crisis response adaptations require new protocols for managing psychiatric emergencies when participants may be in remote locations. This includes knowing participants' locations, emergency contacts, and local resources.

Continuity planning addresses how to maintain therapeutic relationships when technology fails, internet access is interrupted, or other technical problems interfere with consistent contact.

David initially struggled with the online group format because he felt less connected to the facilitator and other members compared to his previous in-person therapy experiences. The facilitator addressed this by scheduling brief individual check-ins between group sessions and using breakout rooms for smaller group interactions.

The facilitator also adapted her communication style for online delivery by being more explicit about emotional responses she was observing, asking more direct questions about participants' experiences, and using chat functions to provide additional support and encouragement.

Over time, David developed strong therapeutic relationships with both the facilitator and group members despite the online format. He appreciated the convenience and reduced social anxiety that came with participating from home while still receiving the benefits of group connection and support.

Hybrid Model Development

Combining in-person and online elements creates hybrid treatment models that can maximize the benefits of both delivery formats while accommodating diverse participant needs and circumstances.

Flexible participation options allow group members to attend some sessions in person and others online based on their schedules, health status, transportation availability, or comfort levels with different formats.

Technology integration in face-to-face sessions might include using apps for real-time feedback, digital tools for skill practice, or online resources for homework and monitoring that extend therapeutic work beyond session boundaries.

Blended group composition includes some members who attend primarily in person, others who participate mainly online, and some who alternate between formats. This requires careful management to ensure all participants feel equally included and valued.

Equipment and infrastructure needs include high-quality cameras, microphones, and internet connectivity in therapy rooms to support smooth integration of remote and in-person participants.

Facilitation skills must adapt to manage both in-person and online participants simultaneously while ensuring that technology enhances rather than dominates the therapeutic process.

Outcome evaluation helps determine which elements of hybrid models are most effective while identifying optimal combinations of in-person and online interventions for different populations and treatment goals.

Maria's group used a hybrid model where core sessions were held in person but supplemental sessions and check-ins were available online. This allowed her to maintain consistent group participation even when childcare issues or transportation problems would have caused absences from in-person sessions.

The hybrid approach also allowed for more frequent contact than would have been possible with only in-person sessions, providing additional support during difficult periods of trauma processing work.

Some group members preferred the in-person format for intensive trauma work but found online sessions helpful for skill practice, check-ins, and maintenance phases of treatment. This flexibility improved overall treatment engagement and outcomes.

Addressing Digital Divide Issues

Technology-based interventions can inadvertently exclude individuals who lack access to devices, reliable internet, or digital literacy skills. Addressing these disparities becomes essential for equitable trauma treatment access.

Access assessment involves understanding participants' technology resources, internet connectivity, and digital skills while identifying barriers that might prevent effective participation in technology-enhanced treatment.

Equipment provision may include lending tablets, smartphones, or computers to participants who lack necessary devices while providing technical support for setup and maintenance.

Internet connectivity support might involve partnering with internet service providers, using mobile hotspots, or providing vouchers for internet access to ensure consistent participation in online treatment components.

Digital literacy training helps participants develop skills needed to use therapeutic technology effectively while building confidence and reducing anxiety about digital participation.

Alternative options ensure that individuals who cannot or prefer not to use technology still have access to effective trauma treatment through traditional in-person services.

Cultural considerations address how different communities relate to technology while ensuring that digital interventions are culturally appropriate and accessible across diverse populations.

Robert initially couldn't participate in online group sessions because he had an older smartphone and unreliable internet service at his apartment. The program provided him with a tablet and connected him with a low-cost internet program, allowing him to access treatment that would otherwise have been unavailable.

The program also provided basic technology training to help Robert learn to use video conferencing software, therapeutic apps, and other digital tools that enhanced his treatment experience.

Addressing these digital divide issues not only improved Robert's treatment outcomes but also demonstrated the program's commitment to serving all community members regardless of their economic circumstances or technology access.

Privacy and Security Considerations

Technology integration in trauma treatment raises significant privacy and security concerns that must be addressed proactively to protect participants' sensitive mental health information and maintain trust in therapeutic relationships.

HIPAA compliance requirements become more complex with technology use, requiring secure platforms, encrypted communications, business associate agreements with technology vendors, and clear policies about data handling and storage.

Informed consent must address technology risks including potential for data breaches, technical failures, and privacy limitations of digital platforms while ensuring participants understand and accept these risks.

Data security measures include encrypted storage, secure transmission, strong authentication protocols, and regular security updates to protect participant information from unauthorized access or cyber attacks.

Home environment privacy considerations address the reality that online therapy occurs in participants' personal spaces where confidentiality may be compromised by family members, roommates, or others who might overhear sessions.

Recording and documentation policies must address when and how online sessions may be recorded, who has access to recordings, how long they're retained, and how they're securely destroyed when no longer needed.

Cross-border considerations arise when participants or therapists are located in different states or countries with varying privacy laws and professional licensing requirements.

Jennifer was initially hesitant to participate in online group sessions because she was concerned about privacy and worried that her personal information might be shared or compromised through technology platforms.

The program addressed her concerns by providing detailed information about their security measures, explaining HIPAA protections, and helping her optimize her home environment for privacy during online sessions.

Clear communication about privacy protections and security measures helped Jennifer feel comfortable with technology use while maintaining her engagement in treatment that significantly improved her trauma recovery outcomes.

Future Directions and Innovation

Technology continues to evolve rapidly, creating new possibilities for trauma treatment delivery while requiring ongoing adaptation and innovation from mental health professionals.

Artificial intelligence integration may eventually provide personalized treatment recommendations, real-time risk assessment, and automated support systems that enhance human therapeutic relationships rather than replacing them.

Biometric monitoring through wearable devices could provide objective data about stress levels, sleep quality, and other physiological markers that inform treatment decisions and track recovery progress.

Social media integration might allow for therapeutic peer support networks while requiring careful attention to privacy, boundaries, and potential for misuse or triggering content.

Gamification elements could make skill practice and homework completion more engaging while providing immediate feedback and motivation for therapeutic work.

Virtual reality advancement will likely create more sophisticated and accessible VR applications for exposure therapy, skills training, and immersive therapeutic experiences.

Predictive analytics may help identify individuals at risk for treatment dropout, symptom worsening, or crisis situations while enabling preventive interventions.

The trauma treatment program began exploring artificial intelligence tools that could provide personalized coping strategy recommendations based on individual symptom patterns and treatment responses, while maintaining human oversight and professional judgment.

Early pilot testing suggested that AI-enhanced treatment could improve outcomes by providing more precisely tailored interventions while freeing therapists to focus on relationship building and complex clinical decision-making.

However, the program maintained strong emphasis on human therapeutic relationships while viewing technology as a tool to enhance rather than replace the fundamental healing that occurs through authentic human connection and professional expertise.

The Human Element in Digital Healing

Technology's greatest contribution to trauma treatment may be its ability to extend and enhance human therapeutic relationships rather than replace them. The most effective digital interventions maintain focus on connection, healing, and growth while using technology to overcome barriers and provide tools that support the fundamentally human process of recovery.

The challenge lies in maintaining the warmth, authenticity, and skilled responsiveness that characterize effective trauma treatment while leveraging technology's capabilities to reach more people, provide better tools, and create more flexible treatment options.

Success requires ongoing attention to both technological competence and therapeutic relationship skills while ensuring that innovation serves healing rather than becoming an end in itself.

Technology Integration Essentials

- Telehealth group therapy requires fundamental adaptations of traditional approaches while maintaining therapeutic factors through platform optimization and engagement strategies
- Digital tools for homework and monitoring extend therapeutic work beyond sessions while providing real-time data that informs treatment planning
- Virtual reality applications offer controlled exposure experiences and skills practice environments that enhance traditional trauma treatment approaches
- App-based interventions must be carefully selected and integrated to ensure they complement rather than replace human therapeutic relationships
- Maintaining therapeutic alliance remotely requires enhanced presence skills and adapted communication techniques for digital environments

- Addressing digital divide issues ensures equitable access to technology-enhanced treatment across diverse populations and economic circumstances

Chapter 20: Therapist Self-Care and Secondary Trauma Prevention

The wounded healer walks a narrow path between empathy and overwhelm, between professional competence and personal vulnerability. Working with trauma survivors requires opening your heart to stories of human suffering while maintaining the emotional stability needed to provide effective treatment. This balance becomes even more challenging in group settings where multiple trauma narratives intersect, creating environments where secondary trauma can accumulate rapidly if clinicians lack adequate protection and support.

Secondary trauma isn't a sign of weakness or incompetence—it's an occupational hazard that affects even the most skilled and experienced trauma therapists. Recognizing this reality while developing effective prevention and treatment strategies becomes essential for both professional effectiveness and personal wellbeing.

Recognizing Vicarious Trauma Symptoms

Secondary trauma often develops gradually, making it difficult to recognize until symptoms become severe enough to interfere with professional effectiveness or personal functioning. Early recognition allows for intervention before problems become entrenched or lead to burnout and career changes.

Intrusive symptoms may include unwanted thoughts about clients' traumatic experiences, nightmares containing elements from clients' stories, intrusive images related to trauma narratives shared in therapy, or preoccupation with clients' safety and wellbeing during personal time.

Avoidance behaviors might involve dreading certain clients or types of trauma content, avoiding social situations that might trigger thoughts about work, emotionally distancing from clients as protection against overwhelming material, or procrastinating on documentation or treatment planning related to difficult cases.

Negative cognitive changes include developing cynical worldviews, losing faith in human goodness or life meaning, becoming preoccupied with danger and vulnerability, or experiencing hopelessness about clients' recovery potential or societal problems.

Mood and anxiety symptoms often present as increased irritability, sadness, or anxiety that seems disproportionate to personal life circumstances. These symptoms may be accompanied by guilt about clients' suffering, anger about injustice and trauma prevalence, or numbness and emotional withdrawal as protective mechanisms.

Physical symptoms can include chronic fatigue, headaches, gastrointestinal problems, sleep disturbances, or other somatic manifestations of chronic stress exposure. These physical symptoms often mirror those experienced by trauma survivors themselves.

Relationship impacts may involve increased conflict with family members, social withdrawal, difficulty maintaining friendships, or problems with intimacy and emotional availability in personal relationships.

Dr. Martinez, a psychologist facilitating multiple trauma groups, began noticing that she was having difficulty sleeping and found herself checking news obsessively, looking for stories about violence and trauma. She realized she had become hypervigilant about her own children's safety and was having intrusive thoughts about her clients' traumatic experiences during family time.

Her recognition of these symptoms led to consultation with a colleague who helped her identify that she was experiencing secondary trauma from her intensive trauma group work. This recognition allowed her to implement self-care strategies before her symptoms worsened or began affecting her clinical effectiveness.

The early intervention included reducing her caseload temporarily, seeking her own therapy to process secondary trauma reactions, and implementing daily mindfulness practices to help separate work and personal life more effectively.

Personal Therapy and Supervision Requirements

Working with trauma requires ongoing attention to one's own psychological wellbeing through both personal therapy and professional supervision. These supports provide essential outlets for processing difficult material while maintaining professional competence and personal resilience.

Personal therapy benefits include providing safe space to process reactions to clients' trauma material, addressing personal trauma history that might interfere with clinical effectiveness, maintaining emotional balance and resilience, and modeling healthy help-seeking behavior for clients.

Therapy timing considerations may include seeking therapy before beginning trauma work, during particularly challenging periods, or as ongoing maintenance to prevent problems from developing. Some therapists benefit from consistent ongoing therapy while others prefer episodic treatment during difficult periods.

Supervision requirements should include regular discussion of challenging cases, processing of emotional reactions to client material, consultation about treatment decisions, and attention to therapist wellbeing and functioning.

Group supervision benefits provide opportunities to learn from colleagues' experiences while normalizing the challenges of trauma work through shared discussion and mutual support.

Peer consultation offers informal opportunities to discuss difficult cases, share resources and strategies, and maintain connection with colleagues who understand the unique challenges of trauma work.

Professional development through training, workshops, and conferences helps maintain competence while providing perspective on one's own work and access to new approaches and resources.

Lisa, a clinical social worker new to trauma group work, initially felt that seeking her own therapy would be admitting professional incompetence. However, her supervisor helped her understand that personal therapy was an ethical responsibility rather than a professional weakness.

Her personal therapy helped her process her own childhood experiences of family violence that had motivated her interest in trauma work but also created vulnerability to secondary trauma when working with similar cases.

The therapy provided essential support during her first year of trauma group facilitation while helping her develop the self-awareness and emotional regulation skills necessary for effective trauma treatment.

Mindfulness and Resilience Practices

Regular mindfulness and resilience practices provide ongoing protection against secondary trauma while building capacity for sustained effectiveness in trauma work. These practices must be personally meaningful and practically sustainable rather than adding additional stress to already demanding schedules.

Mindfulness meditation practices help develop present-moment awareness that can interrupt rumination about clients' trauma stories while building capacity for emotional regulation and stress management.

Body-based practices including yoga, tai chi, or other movement disciplines help maintain physical health while providing outlets for stress and tension that accumulate through trauma work.

Breathing exercises provide immediately accessible tools for managing stress responses during and after difficult sessions while building overall nervous system resilience.

Grounding techniques help maintain connection to present-moment reality when immersed in clients' trauma narratives, preventing excessive identification or emotional overwhelm.

Loving-kindness meditation specifically addresses the emotional depletion that can result from constant exposure to human suffering by cultivating compassion for self and others.

Nature connection through outdoor activities, gardening, or simply spending time in natural environments provides restoration and perspective that counteracts the intensity of trauma work.

Michael, a licensed professional counselor, developed a daily practice that included 20 minutes of morning meditation, a brief walk during his lunch break, and evening yoga practice. These practices helped him maintain emotional balance while working with multiple trauma groups.

He found that the mindfulness practices were particularly helpful for managing the transition between sessions, allowing him to clear his emotional state before seeing the next client while maintaining appropriate empathy and engagement.

The consistency of his practice proved more important than the specific techniques used, as the regular self-care time helped him maintain perspective and resilience even during particularly challenging periods.

Professional Boundaries and Burnout Prevention

Clear professional boundaries protect both therapists and clients while preventing the emotional overwhelm that can lead to burnout and secondary trauma. These boundaries must be maintained consistently while remaining flexible enough to provide effective clinical care.

Emotional boundaries involve maintaining appropriate emotional distance from clients while remaining empathetically engaged. This includes avoiding over-identification with clients, taking responsibility for clients' emotions or outcomes, or allowing clients' trauma to dominate personal emotional life.

Time boundaries include starting and ending sessions on time, limiting availability for crisis calls to reasonable hours, taking lunch breaks, and maintaining separation between work and personal time.

Physical boundaries involve maintaining appropriate physical contact policies, creating comfortable office environments that feel safe for both therapists and clients, and paying attention to personal safety considerations.

Information boundaries include maintaining confidentiality, avoiding inappropriate personal disclosure, and limiting discussion of client information to professional contexts with appropriate individuals.

Responsibility boundaries involve clarifying what therapists can and cannot control while avoiding taking responsibility for clients' choices, life circumstances, or treatment outcomes beyond professional competence and scope.

Caseload management includes maintaining reasonable numbers of clients, balancing difficult cases with less challenging ones, and advocating for sustainable working conditions within employment settings.

Sarah, a therapist working in a community mental health center, found that her caseload of trauma clients had grown to unsustainable levels as word spread about her effectiveness with trauma treatment. She began working longer hours, taking crisis calls at home, and worrying constantly about her clients' wellbeing.

Her recognition that these boundary violations were contributing to her own distress led to difficult conversations with her supervisor about caseload management and agency expectations for availability and responsiveness.

The boundary clarification included establishing specific hours for crisis availability, negotiating a more balanced caseload that included some less intensive cases, and developing better systems for colleague coverage during vacations and time off.

Building Sustainable Trauma Practices

Sustainability in trauma work requires intentional attention to both individual self-care and systemic factors that support or interfere with therapist wellbeing. This sustainability planning helps prevent burnout while maintaining high-quality treatment for clients.

Career pacing involves planning for the long-term demands of trauma work by balancing intensive periods with recovery time, varying types of clinical work, and developing diverse professional interests and skills.

Workplace advocacy includes working to improve organizational policies and practices that support therapist wellbeing such as reasonable caseloads, adequate supervision, professional development opportunities, and trauma-informed workplace policies.

Financial planning addresses the reality that trauma work can be emotionally demanding while often being less financially rewarding than other specialties, requiring careful attention to student loans, retirement planning, and financial security.

Professional community involvement provides ongoing connection with colleagues who understand trauma work challenges while offering opportunities for learning, collaboration, and mutual support.

Meaning-making practices help maintain perspective on the importance and value of trauma work during difficult periods by connecting daily clinical activities with broader purposes and values.

Exit strategy planning involves recognizing when trauma work may no longer be sustainable and developing alternative career paths that utilize trauma expertise in different contexts such as training, supervision, or consultation.

Robert, a trauma therapist with 15 years of experience, began experiencing increasing cynicism and emotional exhaustion despite his commitment to trauma work. His sustainability planning included reducing his trauma group caseload by 25% while adding supervision and training responsibilities that kept him connected to trauma work in less intensive ways.

He also negotiated with his employer to provide training for other therapists interested in trauma work, creating a more sustainable career path that utilized his expertise while reducing his direct exposure to traumatic material.

These changes allowed him to continue contributing to trauma treatment field while maintaining his own wellbeing and preventing complete burnout that might have ended his trauma work career entirely.

Organizational Support Systems

Individual self-care efforts are necessary but insufficient for preventing secondary trauma and burnout. Organizational support systems provide essential infrastructure for maintaining therapist wellbeing while delivering effective trauma treatment services.

Administrative support includes reasonable caseloads, adequate time for documentation and treatment planning, flexible scheduling that accommodates the intensity of trauma work, and administrative assistance that reduces non-clinical burdens on therapists.

Clinical supervision should be ongoing, specialized for trauma work, and focused on both clinical effectiveness and therapist wellbeing. Supervisors should be trained in recognizing and addressing secondary trauma while providing appropriate support and guidance.

Peer support programs create formal and informal opportunities for therapists to support each other through difficult cases, share resources and strategies, and maintain connection with colleagues who understand the unique challenges of trauma work.

Training and development opportunities help therapists maintain competence while providing perspective on their work and access to new approaches that might reduce stress or increase effectiveness.

Employee assistance programs provide access to mental health services, crisis support, and other resources that support therapist wellbeing while recognizing that trauma therapists may need additional support beyond what's required for other clinical specialties.

Workload management systems monitor therapist stress levels, case complexity, and workload balance while making adjustments to prevent overwhelm and maintain sustainable practice conditions.

The community mental health center where Maria worked implemented a comprehensive secondary trauma prevention program that included monthly trauma consultation groups, reduced caseloads for therapists carrying high proportions of trauma cases, and mandatory self-care planning as part of annual performance reviews.

The program also provided funding for therapists to attend trauma conferences and training while offering flexible scheduling that allowed for recovery time after particularly difficult cases or periods.

These organizational supports significantly reduced staff turnover in trauma services while improving job satisfaction and clinical effectiveness among trauma therapists.

Team-Based Care Models

Distributing the emotional burden of trauma work across teams rather than relying on individual therapists can provide better client care while reducing secondary trauma risk for any single provider.

Co-therapy models allow therapists to share the emotional burden of intensive trauma cases while providing mutual support and consultation during sessions. This model can be particularly helpful for complex cases or group therapy work.

Multidisciplinary teams include psychiatrists, social workers, case managers, and other professionals who can share responsibility for different aspects of client care while reducing the burden on any single provider.

Consultation models provide access to specialized expertise for complex cases while offering support and perspective for treating therapists who might otherwise feel isolated or overwhelmed.

Shared caseload approaches allow multiple therapists to work with the same clients in different capacities, providing continuity of care while preventing over-attachment or excessive responsibility for individual outcomes.

Peer counselor integration includes individuals with lived experience of trauma who can provide unique support and perspective while reducing the burden on professional staff for some aspects of care.

Crisis team approaches provide specialized response to psychiatric emergencies while preventing individual therapists from carrying excessive responsibility for client safety and crisis management.

Jennifer participated in a co-therapy model for her most challenging trauma groups, working with a colleague to facilitate sessions and share the emotional burden of intensive trauma processing work. The co-therapy relationship provided ongoing consultation and support while improving the quality of treatment through dual perspectives and skills.

The model also provided natural coverage for vacations and sick days while ensuring continuity of care for group members who might otherwise have experienced treatment disruptions.

Both therapists reported feeling more supported and less emotionally depleted when working in the co-therapy model compared to their previous experiences facilitating trauma groups alone.

Recovery and Renewal Strategies

Even with excellent prevention strategies, trauma therapists may occasionally experience secondary trauma symptoms that require active intervention and recovery support. Recognition and treatment of these symptoms prevents long-term problems while maintaining professional effectiveness.

Early intervention involves recognizing secondary trauma symptoms quickly while seeking appropriate support before problems become severe or entrenched. This might include temporary caseload reductions, increased supervision, or personal therapy.

Treatment approaches for secondary trauma may include individual therapy using trauma-specific treatments, EMDR for therapists' own trauma responses, or group therapy with other trauma professionals who understand the unique challenges of this work.

Recovery planning includes specific strategies for healing from secondary trauma while making necessary changes in work practices to prevent recurrence. This planning should address both immediate symptom relief and long-term prevention strategies.

Career evaluation may be necessary to determine if trauma work remains sustainable or if alternative career paths might better support long-term wellbeing while utilizing trauma expertise in different ways.

Professional identity integration helps therapists understand secondary trauma as an occupational hazard rather than personal failure while maintaining commitment to trauma work when appropriate.

Return to work planning ensures that therapists are adequately recovered before resuming full trauma caseloads while implementing necessary changes to prevent future problems.

David experienced significant secondary trauma symptoms after facilitating a group for combat veterans that included particularly graphic trauma processing over several months. His symptoms included intrusive thoughts about veterans' combat experiences, nightmares, and increased anxiety about violence and safety.

His recovery included temporary reduction of his trauma caseload, personal therapy using EMDR to process his secondary trauma reactions, and consultation with an expert in therapist secondary trauma treatment.

The recovery process took several months but allowed David to return to trauma work with better self-awareness, improved self-care strategies, and realistic understanding of his limits and vulnerabilities.

Professional Growth Through Adversity

Secondary trauma and burnout, while challenging, can also provide opportunities for professional growth, increased self-awareness, and deeper understanding of trauma's impact on both survivors and helpers.

Increased empathy for clients often results from therapists' own experiences of trauma symptoms, creating deeper understanding and more authentic therapeutic relationships.

Enhanced self-awareness about personal vulnerabilities, triggers, and needs can improve both professional effectiveness and personal wellbeing while providing insights that benefit client care.

Improved boundaries often develop as therapists learn from experiences of over-involvement or emotional overwhelm, leading to more sustainable practice patterns and better client outcomes.

Career clarification may result from difficult periods that help therapists understand their strengths, limitations, and preferences while making informed decisions about professional development and career paths.

Teaching and mentoring opportunities often emerge as experienced therapists share their knowledge about secondary trauma prevention and recovery with colleagues, contributing to improved field practices.

Research and advocacy interests may develop as therapists recognize the need for better support systems, prevention strategies, or treatment approaches for trauma professionals.

Lisa's experience of secondary trauma led to her development of expertise in therapist self-care and resilience, eventually becoming a sought-after trainer and consultant who helped other organizations develop secondary trauma prevention programs.

Her personal experience of recovery from secondary trauma provided authenticity and credibility in her training work while allowing her to contribute to improved standards of care for trauma therapists throughout her region.

The challenging experience ultimately enhanced rather than limited her career while providing valuable perspective and expertise that benefited countless other trauma professionals.

The Sacred Work of Healing

Trauma therapy represents sacred work—accompanying others through their darkest moments while witnessing their courage and resilience in the face of overwhelming experiences. This work requires enormous emotional strength while offering profound rewards through participation in human healing and transformation.

The key to sustainability lies in recognizing both the privileges and responsibilities of this work while maintaining the self-awareness and self-care necessary to continue serving others effectively over time.

Professional longevity in trauma work requires balance between empathy and boundaries, between engagement and self-protection, between professional competence and personal vulnerability. This balance is never perfect but must be continually adjusted based on changing circumstances and growing self-awareness.

Professional Sustainability Principles

- Recognizing vicarious trauma symptoms early allows for intervention before problems become severe or interfere with professional effectiveness
- Personal therapy and supervision provide essential outlets for processing difficult material while maintaining professional competence and resilience
- Mindfulness and resilience practices offer ongoing protection against secondary trauma while building capacity for sustained effectiveness
- Professional boundaries prevent emotional overwhelm while maintaining appropriate therapeutic engagement and empathy
- Building sustainable practices requires attention to both individual self-care and systemic factors that support therapist wellbeing
- Organizational support systems provide essential infrastructure for maintaining therapist wellbeing while delivering effective trauma treatment services

Chapter 21: Supervision and Training Models

Teaching someone to hold space for human suffering while maintaining professional competence and personal wellbeing represents one of the most complex challenges in mental health education. Trauma group therapy supervision extends beyond traditional clinical oversight to include specialized skills in group dynamics, complex trauma presentations, crisis management, and the unique challenges of witnessing multiple trauma narratives simultaneously.

The supervisor becomes both teacher and protector—guiding the development of clinical skills while monitoring for secondary trauma, modeling healthy boundaries while encouraging appropriate risk-taking, and building competence while maintaining humility about the profound responsibility of trauma work.

Training Requirements and Competency Standards

Trauma group therapy requires specialized competencies that build upon but extend far beyond general therapy skills. These competencies must be clearly defined, systematically developed, and rigorously assessed to ensure both client safety and therapist effectiveness.

Foundational knowledge requirements include understanding of trauma theory and research, familiarity with various trauma treatment modalities, knowledge of group dynamics and therapeutic factors, and awareness of cultural factors that influence trauma presentation and treatment response.

Clinical skill competencies encompass individual trauma assessment and treatment, group facilitation abilities, crisis intervention skills, and capacity to work with complex presentations including dissociation, substance abuse, and personality disorders.

Specialized trauma knowledge involves understanding different trauma types (developmental, combat, sexual, medical, cultural), trauma's impact on various populations, and evidence-based treatments for complex trauma presentations.

Group-specific skills include ability to manage group dynamics, facilitate interpersonal learning, handle conflict and crisis in group settings, and balance individual needs with group process requirements.

Ethical competencies cover confidentiality in group settings, informed consent for group participation, mandatory reporting requirements, and boundary management with multiple clients simultaneously.

Supervision and training standards should specify minimum hours of didactic training, supervised clinical experience, personal therapy requirements, and ongoing education necessary for competent trauma group practice.

Sarah, a doctoral psychology student, completed a year-long trauma therapy training program that included 40 hours of didactic instruction, 200 hours of supervised clinical experience with trauma clients, participation in weekly group supervision focused on trauma cases, and her own personal therapy to address potential secondary trauma issues.

Her competency evaluation included written examination of trauma theory and evidence-based treatments, live observation of therapy sessions with feedback, case presentation demonstrating clinical reasoning and treatment planning skills, and self-assessment of readiness for independent practice.

The comprehensive training prepared her for the complexity of trauma work while building confidence in her ability to provide effective treatment and recognize when additional consultation or referral might be necessary.

Live Supervision and Consultation Models

Real-time supervision provides immediate guidance during challenging clinical situations while offering learning opportunities that cannot be replicated through post-session consultation alone.

Co-therapy supervision involves experienced supervisors participating directly in group sessions as co-facilitators, providing modeling of advanced skills while offering immediate consultation and support when difficult situations arise.

Observation-based supervision uses one-way mirrors, video technology, or in-room observation to allow supervisors to witness sessions directly while providing feedback and guidance based on actual clinical interactions rather than supervisee reports.

Phone or text consultation during sessions allows supervisees to access immediate guidance when facing challenging situations, providing safety and support while building confidence in handling difficult clinical scenarios.

Group supervision models bring together multiple supervisees to observe and discuss live or recorded sessions, providing diverse perspectives while normalizing the challenges of trauma work through shared learning experiences.

Peer consultation pairs supervisees with more experienced colleagues who provide ongoing support and guidance while sharing responsibility for difficult cases and clinical decisions.

Crisis consultation provides immediate access to specialized expertise when psychiatric emergencies arise, ensuring appropriate response while providing learning opportunities about crisis management.

Michael, a new trauma therapist, participated in a co-therapy supervision model where his supervisor joined him as co-facilitator for his first trauma group. The supervisor provided real-time modeling of advanced skills while offering immediate support during difficult moments.

When one group member became suicidal during a session, the supervisor was able to demonstrate crisis assessment and intervention skills while ensuring appropriate safety measures were implemented. This live learning experience provided invaluable training that could not have been achieved through discussion alone.

The co-therapy model gradually shifted to observation-based supervision as Michael developed competence, with the supervisor eventually transitioning to post-session consultation as he demonstrated readiness for independent practice.

Video Review and Feedback Processes

Video review provides powerful learning opportunities by allowing detailed analysis of clinical interactions while offering multiple perspectives on therapeutic process and technique refinement.

Video selection strategies involve choosing segments that highlight specific learning objectives, challenging clinical situations, or examples of effective interventions while maintaining client confidentiality and obtaining appropriate consent.

Structured review processes provide frameworks for analyzing video content including attention to therapeutic alliance, intervention effectiveness, group dynamics, and therapist use of self while maintaining focus on learning rather than evaluation.

Feedback delivery skills for supervisors include providing balanced feedback that acknowledges strengths while addressing areas for improvement, offering specific suggestions for technique refinement, and maintaining supportive relationships that encourage continued learning.

Self-assessment integration helps supervisees develop capacity for objective self-evaluation by reviewing their own video sessions while identifying strengths, areas for improvement, and questions for supervisor consultation.

Group review sessions allow multiple supervisees to learn from each other's cases while providing diverse perspectives on clinical challenges and intervention strategies.

Technical considerations include video quality requirements, storage and security protocols, client consent procedures, and equipment needs for effective video review supervision.

Jennifer participated in weekly video review supervision where she and her supervisor watched selected segments from her trauma group sessions while discussing clinical decisions, intervention choices, and group dynamics that might not have been apparent during the actual sessions.

The video review helped her recognize subtle patterns in group member interactions, identify moments when her interventions were particularly effective or ineffective, and develop greater awareness of her own therapeutic style and impact on group process.

The detailed analysis possible through video review accelerated her learning while building confidence in her clinical skills and judgment through objective feedback about her actual therapeutic work.

Ethical Considerations in Supervision

Supervision of trauma group therapy involves complex ethical considerations that extend beyond traditional individual therapy supervision to include group confidentiality, multiple client relationships, and the unique vulnerabilities created by trauma work.

Informed consent for supervision must address video recording, case discussion in supervision, supervisor access to client information, and limits of confidentiality when multiple clients are involved in group treatment.

Confidentiality management becomes complex with multiple clients whose information may be discussed in supervision while maintaining privacy protection and appropriate boundaries around information sharing.

Dual relationship issues may arise when supervisors have previous relationships with clients, when supervision occurs in small communities where multiple relationships are unavoidable, or when training programs include personal therapy requirements.

Competence boundaries require clear understanding of supervisor qualifications, supervisee skill levels, and appropriate limits on independent practice while ensuring adequate oversight and support.

Crisis responsibility involves clear agreements about supervisor availability, emergency consultation procedures, and responsibility distribution between supervisors and supervisees when client safety issues arise.

Documentation requirements include supervision records, competency assessments, client safety issues, and treatment planning decisions while protecting client confidentiality and maintaining appropriate professional boundaries.

David's supervision relationship included detailed discussion of ethical boundaries when one of his group members was the sister of a colleague at his workplace. The supervision addressed potential confidentiality complications, ways to manage dual relationship issues, and appropriate consultation when conflicts of interest might arise.

The ethical planning included clear agreements about information sharing, consultation procedures when ethical dilemmas arose, and steps to take if the dual relationship became problematic for either the client or the therapeutic relationship.

This proactive ethical planning prevented problems while providing valuable learning about the complex ethical issues that commonly arise in trauma group work, particularly in smaller communities where multiple relationships are common.

Building Organizational Support Systems

Effective supervision requires organizational support that goes beyond individual supervisor-supervisee relationships to include systemic structures that promote learning, safety, and professional development.

Administrative support includes adequate time allocation for supervision, appropriate caseload management, flexible scheduling that accommodates supervision needs, and administrative recognition of supervision importance for both learning and client safety.

Supervision training for experienced clinicians who are developing supervision skills ensures that supervisors have necessary knowledge and abilities to provide effective oversight and guidance for trauma group work.

Peer support networks connect supervisees with colleagues facing similar challenges while providing informal consultation and mutual support that supplements formal supervision relationships.

Continuing education opportunities help both supervisors and supervisees stay current with developments in trauma treatment while building specialized knowledge and skills needed for effective practice.

Quality assurance systems monitor supervision effectiveness while ensuring that training standards are met and client safety is maintained throughout the learning process.

Career development planning helps supervisees understand professional pathways in trauma work while providing guidance about specialization opportunities, advanced training, and professional goals.

The community mental health agency where Lisa worked implemented a comprehensive supervision support system that included weekly individual supervision, monthly group consultation meetings, quarterly training workshops, and annual professional development planning for all trauma therapists.

Supervisors received their own training and consultation about effective supervision practices while participating in a supervisor support group that addressed the unique challenges of supervising trauma work.

The organizational support significantly improved both the quality of supervision and the retention of trauma therapists while building a culture of learning and professional development that attracted high-quality staff and improved client outcomes.

Developmental Supervision Models

Supervision needs change as supervisees develop competence, requiring flexible approaches that match supervision intensity and focus to individual learning needs and skill levels.

Beginning practitioner supervision provides intensive oversight with frequent contact, detailed case review, crisis consultation availability, and extensive skill building through modeling and direct instruction.

Intermediate supervision reduces intensity while maintaining regular contact, focuses on skill refinement and clinical judgment development, and increases supervisee autonomy while providing consultation for complex cases.

Advanced supervision emphasizes consultation rather than oversight, addresses specialized skills and complex cases, and supports professional development and potential supervision training for experienced practitioners.

Competency-based progression uses objective criteria to determine supervision level changes rather than relying solely on time-based advancement, ensuring that supervisees demonstrate necessary skills before receiving increased autonomy.

Individual adaptation recognizes that different supervisees may progress at different rates while requiring varying types of support and guidance based on their learning styles, previous experience, and current skill levels.

Crisis response protocols ensure appropriate supervision intensity during difficult periods regardless of supervisee's usual developmental level, providing additional support when challenging cases or personal issues affect clinical effectiveness.

Robert's supervision evolved from intensive weekly individual meetings with detailed case review during his first year to monthly consultation sessions focused on complex cases and professional development during his third year of trauma group work.

His supervisor used specific competency benchmarks to guide supervision level changes including independent crisis management, effective group facilitation skills, appropriate consultation seeking, and demonstrated ability to maintain professional boundaries.

The developmental approach allowed for individualized supervision that matched his learning needs while ensuring appropriate oversight and support throughout his professional development as a trauma group therapist.

Specialized Training Tracks

Different populations and trauma presentations may require specialized training tracks that build upon foundational trauma group skills while developing expertise in specific areas.

Population-specific training focuses on particular groups such as military veterans, first responders, refugees, or LGBTQ+ individuals while addressing unique trauma presentations, cultural considerations, and specialized intervention approaches.

Trauma-type specialization develops expertise in specific trauma categories such as sexual trauma, childhood abuse, medical trauma, or disaster response while building knowledge of evidence-based treatments for these presentations.

Modality-specific training focuses on particular treatment approaches such as EMDR, somatic therapies, expressive arts, or cognitive-behavioral treatments while integrating these approaches with group therapy principles.

Setting-specific training addresses unique considerations for different practice environments such as inpatient units, residential treatment, community mental health, or private practice while adapting skills to different organizational contexts.

Advanced practice training prepares experienced therapists for supervision, training, program development, or research roles while building leadership skills and advanced clinical expertise.

Cultural competency tracks develop specialized knowledge about working with specific cultural groups while addressing historical trauma, cultural healing practices, and systemic oppression factors that affect treatment.

Maria completed a specialized training track in refugee trauma that included cultural competency development, interpreter work skills, understanding of pre-migration trauma and post-migration stressors, and coordination with legal and social service providers.

The specialized training prepared her to work effectively with refugee populations while building expertise that made her a valuable resource for colleagues and organizations serving these communities.

Her specialized knowledge also led to consultation opportunities, training provision for other therapists, and program development work that expanded services for refugee trauma survivors in her region.

Technology Integration in Supervision

Technology increasingly supports supervision processes while providing new opportunities for learning, consultation, and professional development that transcend geographic limitations and scheduling constraints.

Video conferencing supervision allows for real-time consultation regardless of geographic location while providing access to specialized supervisors who might not be available locally.

Digital platforms for case presentation, resource sharing, and supervision documentation improve efficiency while creating searchable records of supervision activities and learning progress.

Remote session observation through secure video technology allows supervisors to observe sessions from distant locations while providing immediate consultation and feedback.

Online training modules supplement in-person supervision with standardized learning materials, competency assessments, and specialized content that may not be available through local resources.

Virtual reality training applications may eventually provide standardized training scenarios for crisis management, group facilitation skills, and other competencies that require practice in safe environments.

AI-enhanced supervision might eventually provide automated analysis of therapy sessions, risk assessment, and personalized training recommendations while maintaining human oversight and clinical judgment.

Jennifer participated in a hybrid supervision model that combined weekly in-person meetings with her supervisor and monthly video conferencing sessions with a nationally recognized trauma expert who provided specialized consultation for complex cases.

The technology integration allowed her to access expertise that would not have been available in her rural location while maintaining the personal connection and immediate support provided by her local supervisor.

The hybrid model provided broader learning opportunities while demonstrating how technology could enhance rather than replace traditional supervision relationships and methods.

Evaluation and Outcome Assessment

Systematic evaluation of supervision effectiveness ensures that training goals are met while identifying areas for improvement in both individual supervision relationships and overall training programs.

Competency assessment uses objective criteria to evaluate supervisee skill development while providing feedback about areas of strength and continued learning needs.

Supervision satisfaction measures assess both supervisor and supervisee satisfaction with the supervision relationship while identifying factors that contribute to effective learning partnerships.

Client outcome tracking examines whether supervised therapists achieve positive treatment outcomes while identifying supervision factors that may influence clinical effectiveness.

Program evaluation assesses overall training program effectiveness while identifying successful components and areas needing improvement or modification.

Long-term follow-up tracks supervisee career development, continued competence, and professional satisfaction to evaluate the lasting impact of supervision and training experiences.

Continuous improvement processes use evaluation data to refine supervision approaches, training content, and program structure while ensuring that training remains current and effective.

The trauma training program conducted annual evaluation that included competency assessments for all supervisees, satisfaction surveys for both supervisors and supervisees, and tracking of client outcomes for supervised therapists.

The evaluation data revealed that supervisees who received live supervision and video review showed faster skill development and better client outcomes compared to those receiving only traditional post-session supervision.

This finding led to program modifications that increased the use of live supervision and video review while demonstrating the value of these intensive supervision approaches for trauma therapy training.

Building Future Leaders

Effective supervision not only develops individual competence but also prepares future supervisors, trainers, and leaders who will carry forward the knowledge and values of ethical, effective trauma treatment.

Leadership development includes opportunities for supervisees to develop training skills, program development abilities, and professional leadership capacities while building expertise in trauma treatment.

Mentorship relationships extend beyond formal supervision to include ongoing professional guidance, career development support, and connection to professional networks and opportunities.

Research integration exposes supervisees to current research while encouraging participation in outcome evaluation, program development, and potential research activities that advance the field.

Professional identity development helps supervisees understand their role in the broader trauma treatment field while building commitment to ethical practice, continued learning, and service to trauma survivors.

Succession planning ensures continuity of supervision and training resources while developing new supervisors who can maintain and expand trauma treatment services.

David's supervision experience included opportunities to co-facilitate training workshops, participate in program development activities, and eventually provide supervision to newer therapists under his supervisor's guidance.

These leadership development opportunities helped him develop a broader perspective on trauma treatment while building skills that enhanced his career opportunities and contribution to the field.

His transition from supervisee to supervisor demonstrated the success of developmental supervision models that prepare experienced practitioners to become the next generation of trauma treatment leaders and educators.

The Ripple Effect of Excellence

Quality supervision creates ripple effects that extend far beyond individual learning relationships to influence entire organizations, professional communities, and ultimately the trauma survivors who receive treatment from well-trained, well-supported therapists.

Investment in supervision excellence pays dividends through improved client outcomes, reduced therapist burnout, enhanced professional satisfaction, and stronger trauma treatment programs that can serve more people effectively.

The commitment to training excellence reflects recognition that trauma work requires specialized knowledge, ongoing support, and continuous learning to maintain both effectiveness and sustainability over time.

Training Excellence Components

- Training requirements and competency standards ensure systematic development of specialized skills needed for effective trauma group therapy
- Live supervision and consultation models provide immediate guidance while offering learning opportunities unavailable through traditional post-session consultation
- Video review processes allow detailed analysis of clinical interactions while accelerating skill development through objective feedback
- Ethical considerations in supervision address complex confidentiality and relationship issues unique to group therapy supervision
- Organizational support systems provide infrastructure necessary for effective supervision while promoting learning and professional development
- Developmental supervision models adapt intensity and focus to individual learning needs while ensuring appropriate oversight throughout skill development

Chapter 22: Program Development and Implementation

Building a trauma group therapy program from concept to sustainable service requires navigating complex organizational, clinical, and financial challenges while maintaining unwavering focus on the ultimate goal: creating healing opportunities for trauma survivors who might otherwise go without effective treatment. Success demands both visionary leadership and meticulous attention to practical details that can make or break program viability.

The path from initial idea to thriving program is littered with well-intentioned efforts that failed due to inadequate planning, insufficient resources, or unrealistic expectations about implementation challenges. Learning from these failures while building on successful models provides the foundation for developing programs that can serve trauma survivors effectively while remaining financially sustainable.

Needs Assessment and Program Design

Effective program development begins with thorough understanding of community needs, available resources, and service gaps that the new program might address. This assessment provides the foundation for all subsequent planning while ensuring that program design matches actual rather than assumed needs.

Community trauma epidemiology involves understanding local trauma prevalence, types of trauma most common in the area, demographic characteristics of trauma survivors, and current service utilization patterns that indicate unmet needs.

Existing service mapping identifies current trauma treatment resources including individual therapy, other group programs, inpatient services, crisis resources, and specialized programs while identifying gaps that might be addressed through new program development.

Stakeholder analysis examines key individuals and organizations that might support or resist program development including potential referral sources, funding organizations, competing providers, and community leaders whose support might be essential.

Target population definition specifies which trauma survivors the program will serve including trauma types, severity levels, demographic characteristics, and other inclusion/exclusion criteria that will guide program design and marketing efforts.

Service model development translates needs assessment findings into specific program components including group formats, treatment duration, staffing models, and integration with other services.

Outcome expectations establish realistic goals for program impact including client outcomes, service volume, financial performance, and community benefit that will guide implementation and evaluation efforts.

The community mental health center conducted an extensive needs assessment that revealed high rates of childhood sexual abuse among adult women seeking services but limited specialized treatment options. The assessment identified 200-300 potential clients who might benefit from trauma group services while revealing that individual therapy waitlists exceeded six months.

Stakeholder interviews revealed strong support from local domestic violence organizations, child advocacy centers, and healthcare providers who were seeking referral resources for trauma survivors. However, the assessment also identified concerns from some community members about "stirring up" traumatic memories and potential liability issues.

The needs assessment guided development of a women's trauma group program that specifically addressed childhood sexual abuse while building partnerships with community organizations and addressing community concerns through education and outreach efforts.

Staffing Models and Resource Allocation

Staffing decisions significantly impact both program quality and financial sustainability while determining the types of services that can be offered and the populations that can be served effectively.

Staffing ratios must balance adequate supervision and support with cost-effectiveness while ensuring that groups can operate safely and effectively. Most trauma groups require at least one highly qualified facilitator with backup support for crisis situations.

Qualifications and competencies for staff include specialized trauma training, group therapy experience, crisis intervention skills, and cultural competence for serving diverse populations while maintaining appropriate licensure and credentialization.

Training and development requirements include initial specialized training, ongoing supervision, continuing education, and professional development opportunities that maintain staff competence while building program reputation and staff retention.

Supervision structures provide ongoing clinical oversight, consultation for difficult cases, administrative support, and professional development guidance while ensuring compliance with regulatory requirements and professional standards.

Support staff needs may include intake coordinators, schedulers, data collection staff, and administrative support that allows clinical staff to focus on direct service delivery while maintaining efficient program operation.

Salary and benefit considerations must attract qualified staff while remaining within budget constraints, often requiring creative approaches to compensation including professional development opportunities, flexible scheduling, or unique benefits.

Sarah led the development of a first responder trauma program that required staff with both trauma expertise and credibility with police, fire, and EMS personnel. The staffing model included a program director with both clinical and first responder backgrounds, trauma-trained clinicians with group therapy experience, and peer support specialists who were retired first responders.

The staffing approach addressed the unique cultural competence needed for this population while providing appropriate clinical expertise and administrative support. Salary considerations included recognition that staff with first responder backgrounds might command higher salaries but would also bring unique credibility and effectiveness.

The model also included ongoing training partnerships with first responder organizations and trauma treatment experts to maintain staff competence while building program reputation within first responder communities.

Marketing and Referral Development

Successful programs require effective marketing and referral development strategies that build awareness among potential clients and referral sources while accurately representing program services and capabilities.

Target audience identification includes both potential clients and referral sources such as individual therapists, medical providers, employee assistance programs, legal advocates, and community organizations that serve trauma survivors.

Marketing message development communicates program benefits clearly while addressing potential concerns or misconceptions about trauma group therapy, maintaining sensitivity to trauma survivors' fears and hesitations about seeking treatment.

Referral source cultivation involves building relationships with professionals and organizations likely to refer clients while providing education about trauma group therapy benefits and program-specific features that make referrals appropriate.

Community education helps increase awareness about trauma's prevalence and impact while reducing stigma and encouraging help-seeking behavior among potential clients who might otherwise avoid treatment.

Professional networking through conferences, training events, and professional organizations builds program visibility while establishing credibility with potential referral sources and collaborating organizations.

Outcome dissemination involves sharing program effectiveness data with referral sources and community stakeholders while building evidence base that supports continued referrals and program expansion.

Michael developed a comprehensive marketing strategy for his combat veteran trauma program that included presentations to Veterans Administration staff, partnerships with veteran service organizations, outreach to military family support groups, and collaboration with veteran-owned businesses.

The marketing approach emphasized the program's understanding of military culture, use of evidence-based treatments, and staffing by clinicians with military experience or specialized training. Materials addressed common concerns about confidentiality, career impact, and stigma that prevent many veterans from seeking mental health treatment.

The strategy also included testimonials from program graduates who were willing to share their positive experiences while maintaining appropriate confidentiality and professional boundaries.

Quality Assurance and Fidelity Monitoring

Maintaining program quality and treatment fidelity ensures that clients receive effective services while protecting program reputation and supporting continued funding and referrals.

Treatment protocol development specifies exactly what services will be provided, how they will be delivered, and what outcomes are expected while providing clear guidance for staff about program standards and expectations.

Fidelity monitoring involves regular assessment of whether services are being delivered as intended while identifying deviations that might affect program effectiveness or client safety.

Outcome tracking measures client progress, program effectiveness, and service quality while providing data for program improvement and accountability to funders and stakeholders.

Quality improvement processes use monitoring data to identify problems and implement solutions while continuously refining program operations to enhance effectiveness and efficiency.

Staff performance evaluation ensures that individual staff members are meeting program standards while providing feedback and support for professional development and performance improvement.

External oversight may include accreditation bodies, licensing agencies, funding organizations, or professional consultants who provide objective assessment of program quality and compliance with standards.

Jennifer implemented a comprehensive quality assurance system for her refugee trauma program that included weekly supervision for all staff, monthly review of randomly selected case files, quarterly client satisfaction surveys, and annual program evaluation by external consultants.

The monitoring system identified that interpretation services were sometimes inadequate for complex trauma discussions, leading to program modifications that included specialized interpreter training and additional time allocation for sessions requiring interpretation.

The quality assurance data also revealed that clients who completed the full program showed significant improvement on standardized trauma measures while reporting high satisfaction with services and strong likelihood of recommending the program to others.

Sustainability and Funding Considerations

Long-term program sustainability requires diversified funding sources, efficient operation, and demonstrated value that attracts continued support from multiple stakeholders.

Funding diversification reduces dependence on any single source while providing stability that allows for long-term planning and development. Funding sources might include government grants, private foundations, fee-for-service revenue, donor contributions, and organizational support.

Cost-effectiveness demonstration involves showing that program services provide good value for money invested while comparing costs to alternative service models or to the costs of not providing services.

Revenue generation through fee-for-service billing, training and consultation contracts, or other income-producing activities can supplement grant funding while building program sustainability.

Efficiency optimization involves streamlining operations, reducing unnecessary costs, and maximizing the use of available resources while maintaining service quality and effectiveness.

Stakeholder engagement maintains support from funders, referral sources, and community leaders while building constituencies that will advocate for continued program funding and development.

Strategic planning addresses long-term program development while anticipating funding changes, service evolution, and expansion opportunities that might enhance sustainability.

Robert developed a sustainability plan for his healthcare worker trauma program that included initial foundation funding for program development, fee-for-service revenue from hospital employee assistance programs, training contracts with healthcare organizations, and eventual integration into hospital system budgets.

The plan recognized that initial funding would be needed to demonstrate program effectiveness while building the reputation and relationships necessary for ongoing sustainability through diversified revenue sources.

The sustainability approach also included cost-effectiveness analysis showing that trauma treatment for healthcare workers reduced turnover, sick leave utilization, and worker compensation claims while improving job satisfaction and patient care quality.

Evaluation and Continuous Improvement

Systematic evaluation provides essential feedback about program effectiveness while identifying opportunities for improvement and generating data that supports sustainability and expansion efforts.

Evaluation design specifies what will be measured, how data will be collected, when assessments will occur, and how results will be used while balancing scientific rigor with practical feasibility.

Data collection systems must be efficient and minimally burdensome while capturing meaningful information about client outcomes, program processes, and cost-effectiveness.

Outcome measurement includes both clinical outcomes (symptom reduction, functional improvement) and program outcomes (completion rates, client satisfaction, referral source satisfaction) while tracking both short-term and long-term results.

Process evaluation examines how program services are delivered while identifying strengths and weaknesses in program implementation that might affect client outcomes or operational efficiency.

Stakeholder feedback from clients, staff, referral sources, and funders provides qualitative information about program effectiveness while identifying areas for improvement and development.

Report development communicates evaluation findings to various audiences while demonstrating program value and supporting requests for continued funding and organizational support.

Lisa implemented a comprehensive evaluation system for her first responder trauma program that included pre- and post-treatment assessments of trauma symptoms and job performance, six-month follow-up evaluations, staff satisfaction surveys, and interviews with program participants and their supervisors.

The evaluation data showed significant improvements in trauma symptoms, job satisfaction, and family relationships while demonstrating reduced absenteeism and worker compensation claims among program participants.

The evaluation findings supported successful grant applications for program expansion while providing evidence that convinced additional fire and police departments to contract for program services.

Regulatory and Legal Compliance

Program development must address numerous regulatory requirements and legal considerations that affect both program operation and client safety while ensuring compliance with professional standards and organizational policies.

Licensing requirements for facilities, programs, and individual staff must be understood and maintained while ensuring that all applicable regulations are followed throughout program implementation and operation.

Privacy and confidentiality regulations including HIPAA requirements become complex in group settings while requiring careful attention to information sharing, documentation practices, and technology use.

Informed consent procedures must address group-specific issues including confidentiality limitations, recording policies, crisis procedures, and client rights while ensuring that participants understand what they are agreeing to.

Risk management involves identifying potential liability issues including client safety, staff actions, facility concerns, and documentation requirements while implementing policies and procedures that minimize legal risks.

Professional standards from licensing boards, professional organizations, and accreditation bodies must be incorporated into program policies while ensuring that staff understand and follow applicable ethical guidelines.

Insurance considerations include professional liability coverage, general liability protection, and property insurance while understanding coverage limitations and requirements for trauma-specific programming.

David worked with his organization's legal counsel to ensure that his combat veteran trauma program met all applicable regulatory requirements including state licensing for group therapy programs, federal regulations for serving veterans, and professional standards for trauma treatment.

The compliance process included development of detailed policies and procedures, staff training on regulatory requirements, documentation systems that met various oversight needs, and regular review of compliance status.

The proactive approach to regulatory compliance prevented problems while building credibility with oversight agencies and demonstrating program commitment to maintaining high standards of care.

Technology Integration and Infrastructure

Modern program development must consider technology needs that support both service delivery and program administration while ensuring that technology enhances rather than complicates program operations.

Electronic health records systems must accommodate group therapy documentation while maintaining confidentiality, supporting billing processes, and providing data for evaluation and quality assurance activities.

Communication systems including secure messaging, video conferencing, and client portal access can enhance service delivery while maintaining HIPAA compliance and protecting client privacy.

Data management requires systems for collecting, storing, analyzing, and reporting outcome data while maintaining security and supporting both clinical and administrative needs.

Telehealth capabilities may be essential for serving clients in rural areas, accommodating scheduling conflicts, or providing services during public health emergencies while maintaining service quality and therapeutic relationships.

Security measures protect both client information and program operations from cyber threats while ensuring compliance with healthcare privacy regulations and organizational policies.

Staff training ensures that all team members can use technology effectively while understanding security requirements and troubleshooting common problems that might interfere with service delivery.

Maria integrated technology throughout her refugee trauma program including electronic health records with multi-language capabilities, video conferencing for remote participation, and mobile apps for symptom tracking and crisis support.

The technology integration required significant initial investment and staff training but ultimately improved program efficiency while expanding service accessibility for clients who faced transportation barriers or scheduling conflicts.

The program also partnered with a local technology company to provide donated equipment and technical support while building community relationships that enhanced program sustainability.

Expansion and Replication Planning

Successful programs often face opportunities or pressures to expand services or replicate programming in other locations while maintaining quality and effectiveness that made the original program successful.

Expansion planning considers how to increase service capacity, add new program components, or serve additional populations while maintaining program quality and organizational capacity to support growth.

Replication models specify how program elements can be adapted for different settings, populations, or organizational contexts while maintaining fidelity to core components that drive effectiveness.

Training and consultation services can provide revenue while disseminating effective practices to other organizations and communities that want to develop similar programming.

Quality control becomes more challenging as programs expand while requiring systems that ensure consistent service delivery and outcomes across multiple sites or service components.

Organizational development may be necessary to support expansion while building administrative capacity, supervision structures, and quality assurance systems that can manage increased complexity.

Partnership opportunities with other organizations can facilitate expansion while sharing resources, expertise, and costs associated with program development and implementation.

Robert's first responder program began receiving requests from other communities to help develop similar services, leading to development of a replication model that included training curricula, implementation guides, consultation services, and ongoing support for new programs.

The replication approach generated additional revenue while extending program impact beyond the original community and building a network of similar programs that could share resources and expertise.

The expansion also enhanced the original program's sustainability by diversifying revenue sources while building reputation and credibility that attracted additional funding and partnership opportunities.

Measuring Success and Impact

Program success must be defined clearly and measured systematically while recognizing that different stakeholders may have different definitions of success and different expectations for program outcomes.

Client-level outcomes include symptom reduction, functional improvement, quality of life enhancement, and satisfaction with services while tracking both immediate and long-term results.

Program-level outcomes involve service volume, completion rates, cost-effectiveness, and operational efficiency while demonstrating program contribution to organizational goals and community needs.

System-level impacts might include reduced utilization of crisis services, improved functioning of other service systems, and enhanced community capacity to serve trauma survivors effectively.

Staff outcomes include job satisfaction, professional development, retention rates, and skill enhancement while ensuring that program implementation supports rather than burdens staff wellbeing.

Organizational benefits involve reputation enhancement, revenue generation, mission fulfillment, and strategic positioning while demonstrating program value to organizational leadership and stakeholders.

Community impact includes increased awareness of trauma issues, reduced stigma about mental health treatment, and enhanced capacity to support trauma survivors while building community resilience and resources.

Jennifer's comprehensive evaluation of her healthcare worker trauma program demonstrated significant improvements in participant trauma symptoms and job satisfaction while showing reduced turnover and absenteeism among program participants.

The evaluation also revealed that participating healthcare organizations reported improved workplace culture, reduced worker compensation claims, and enhanced ability to recruit and retain staff in high-stress positions.

These multiple levels of impact data supported successful grant applications while convincing additional healthcare organizations to contract for program services and demonstrating the program's value to multiple stakeholder groups.

The Architecture of Hope

Program development represents an act of faith—believing that systematic planning, adequate resources, and skilled implementation can create opportunities for healing that transform individual lives while strengthening communities' capacity to support trauma survivors.

Success requires balancing visionary thinking with practical problem-solving while maintaining unwavering commitment to the ultimate goal of providing effective trauma treatment to individuals who might otherwise suffer without relief.

The programs that endure and thrive are those that combine clinical excellence with operational sustainability while building communities of support that extend far beyond formal service boundaries.

Program Development Fundamentals

- Needs assessment and program design ensure that services match actual community needs while building on available resources and addressing service gaps
- Staffing models and resource allocation balance quality with cost-effectiveness while ensuring adequate expertise and support for complex trauma treatment
- Marketing and referral development build awareness and relationships while accurately representing program capabilities and addressing potential concerns
- Quality assurance and fidelity monitoring maintain treatment effectiveness while protecting program reputation and supporting continuous improvement
- Sustainability and funding considerations ensure long-term viability through diversified revenue sources and demonstrated value to multiple stakeholders
- Evaluation and continuous improvement provide essential feedback while generating data that supports program development and stakeholder engagement

Chapter 23: Recovery, Integration, and Relapse Prevention

The end of a trauma group marks not the completion of healing but the beginning of a new chapter—one where survivors must take their hard-won insights, newly developed skills, and fragile sense of hope into a world that may not have changed while they were in treatment. This transition from the protected environment of group therapy to independent living requires careful planning, ongoing support, and realistic expectations about the nonlinear nature of recovery.

Graduation represents both achievement and loss. Group members celebrate their progress while grieving the end of relationships that may have provided their first experience of genuine safety and acceptance. The skills they've learned must now be tested in situations far more complex and unpredictable than anything encountered in group sessions.

Graduation Criteria and Transition Planning

Determining readiness for group completion requires balancing objective progress measures with subjective readiness indicators while recognizing that trauma recovery is a lifelong process rather than a destination that can be definitively reached.

Symptom improvement benchmarks provide concrete evidence of therapeutic progress including reduced PTSD symptoms, improved emotional regulation, decreased dissociation, and enhanced daily functioning. However, these measures must be interpreted within individual contexts recognizing that some survivors may never achieve "normal" scores on standardized instruments.

Functional capacity indicators examine whether group members can manage basic life responsibilities including work or school attendance, relationship maintenance, self-care activities, and independent living skills. The goal is functional improvement rather than perfect functioning.

Skills demonstration involves showing that members can use coping strategies learned in group settings to manage triggers, emotional overwhelm, and interpersonal challenges outside the therapy room. This includes both prevention skills and crisis management abilities.

Relationship capacity assessment considers members' ability to maintain healthy boundaries, communicate needs effectively, and engage in mutual relationships rather than one-sided dynamics based on trauma patterns.

Integration indicators involve demonstrating that traumatic experiences have been processed to the point where they no longer dominate daily life while maintaining realistic awareness of ongoing vulnerability and need for continued self-care.

Individual readiness factors recognize that each person's recovery timeline differs based on trauma severity, available resources, co-occurring conditions, and personal circumstances that affect healing capacity.

Maria's graduation criteria included achieving scores in the mild range on PTSD measures, demonstrating consistent use of grounding techniques during triggered states, maintaining stable housing and employment, and developing supportive relationships outside the group. However, her transition planning also acknowledged ongoing vulnerability around anniversary dates and continued need for support during family visits that triggered childhood memories.

The graduation planning process took three months and included gradual reduction in group attendance, development of detailed crisis plans, connection with ongoing individual therapy, and identification of peer support resources. Maria also completed a personal recovery plan that outlined warning signs, coping strategies, and support resources for managing future challenges.

Her transition plan recognized that graduation represented the beginning of independent recovery work rather than the end of healing needs, with clear pathways for accessing additional support if symptoms returned or new challenges emerged.

Maintenance Strategies and Booster Sessions

Maintaining therapeutic gains requires ongoing attention and practice while recognizing that recovery exists on a continuum rather than as a fixed state that can be permanently achieved.

Daily practice routines help integrate coping skills into regular life patterns while maintaining the nervous system regulation and emotional balance developed during group treatment. These routines must be realistic and sustainable rather than burdensome additions to already challenging lives.

Environmental modifications support continued recovery by reducing unnecessary stressors, increasing safety cues, and structuring living situations to promote stability and wellbeing. This might include changes in housing, work situations, or social environments.

Relationship maintenance involves nurturing supportive connections while managing challenging relationships that might trigger trauma responses. This includes both family relationships and friendships developed during and after treatment.

Professional support continuation through individual therapy, psychiatric care, or other professional services provides ongoing resources for managing challenges that arise after group completion while maintaining connection to mental health support systems.

Peer support engagement helps maintain connection with others who understand trauma recovery while providing mutual support and accountability for continued growth and healing.

Booster session scheduling provides planned opportunities to reconnect with group facilitators and potentially other group members while addressing challenges that have emerged since graduation and refreshing skills that may have become less practiced.

Robert's maintenance strategy included daily meditation practice, weekly individual therapy sessions, monthly participation in a veteran support group, and quarterly booster sessions with his trauma group facilitator. He also maintained contact with two other group members who had become close friends during treatment.

His environmental modifications included negotiating flexible work arrangements that reduced stress, creating a home meditation space that supported daily practice, and limiting contact with family members who remained critical and unsupportive of his recovery efforts.

The booster sessions provided opportunities to address new challenges including relationship difficulties, job stress, and anniversary reactions while refreshing skills that had become less practiced since group completion.

Alumni Groups and Peer Support Networks

Former group members often become valuable resources for each other while benefiting from continued connection with others who understand their experiences and support their ongoing recovery efforts.

**Alumni group

formats** might include monthly meetings facilitated by former group leaders, peer-led support groups, social gatherings, or structured activities that maintain connection while providing ongoing mutual support.

Peer mentoring allows group graduates to support newer members or others beginning their recovery journey while reinforcing their own progress and providing opportunities to give back to the community that supported their healing.

Crisis support networks enable former group members to provide mutual support during difficult times while maintaining connections that can prevent isolation and deterioration during challenging periods.

Activity-based connections through exercise groups, creative activities, volunteer work, or other shared interests help maintain relationships while providing positive activities that support continued wellbeing and recovery.

Online communities facilitate ongoing connection for members who may be geographically separated while providing 24-hour access to peer support and encouragement during difficult times.

Advocacy opportunities allow group graduates to become involved in trauma awareness, policy change, or service development while finding meaning and purpose through their recovery experiences.

Jennifer helped establish an alumni group that met monthly for coffee and conversation, providing ongoing connection for members of her women's trauma group. The informal gatherings allowed former group members to share updates, seek advice about challenges, and maintain the supportive relationships that had been central to their healing.

The alumni group also organized annual fundraising events for the community mental health center, providing opportunities for former group members to give back while raising awareness about trauma treatment services in their community.

Several alumni became peer mentors for new group members, sharing their experiences and hope while demonstrating that recovery was possible even after severe trauma experiences.

Relapse Prevention and Crisis Planning

Trauma recovery rarely follows a straight line, and temporary setbacks or symptom increases should be anticipated and planned for rather than viewed as treatment failures or personal inadequacies.

Trigger identification involves recognizing specific situations, emotions, sensations, or anniversaries that tend to activate trauma responses while developing strategies for managing these predictable challenges.

Early warning systems help individuals recognize subtle signs that their emotional state is becoming unstable before full symptom relapse occurs, allowing for early intervention that can prevent more serious deterioration.

Coping strategy hierarchies provide graduated responses to different levels of distress, from mild techniques for everyday stress to intensive interventions for severe symptom episodes or crisis situations.

Support system activation includes clear plans for when and how to seek help from friends, family, professionals, or crisis services while overcoming barriers that might prevent appropriate help-seeking.

Crisis resource identification ensures ready access to emergency services, crisis hotlines, supportive individuals, and safe environments when symptoms become overwhelming or dangerous.

Recovery plan updating recognizes that relapse prevention strategies may need modification as life circumstances change and new challenges emerge while maintaining flexibility and realistic expectations.

David's relapse prevention plan identified job stress, relationship conflicts, and anniversary dates of his combat experiences as primary triggers while outlining specific strategies for managing each type of challenge. His early warning signs included sleep disturbances, increased irritability, and social withdrawal.

His coping strategy hierarchy ranged from daily meditation and exercise for mild stress to individual therapy sessions for moderate difficulties to crisis hotline contact and emergency department visits for severe symptoms or suicidal thoughts.

The plan also included specific instructions for his wife about how to recognize when he needed additional support and how to encourage help-seeking without becoming demanding or controlling.

Long-term Recovery and Post-traumatic Growth

The ultimate goal of trauma treatment extends beyond symptom reduction to include the possibility of post-traumatic growth—positive changes that emerge from the struggle with trauma and the recovery process.

Meaning-making processes help individuals understand their trauma experiences within broader life contexts while finding purposes and significance that transcend the original harm and suffering.

Strength identification involves recognizing personal qualities, abilities, and resources that enabled survival and recovery while building confidence in one's capacity to handle future challenges.

Relationship enhancement includes developing deeper, more authentic connections with others based on increased self-awareness, emotional capacity, and ability to be vulnerable and genuine in relationships.

Spiritual development may involve deepened religious faith, connection with nature, expanded sense of life purpose, or enhanced appreciation for existence and human experience.

Wisdom acquisition encompasses increased understanding of human nature, life priorities, personal values, and what truly matters in living while developing perspective that comes from surviving significant adversity.

Service orientation often emerges as trauma survivors find ways to help others who have experienced similar challenges while contributing to community healing and resilience.

Sarah's post-traumatic growth included deeper appreciation for her relationships with her children, career change from business to social work, and involvement in sexual abuse prevention programs. She described feeling more authentic and purposeful than before her trauma experiences, though she acknowledged ongoing challenges and vulnerabilities.

Her growth also included enhanced emotional capacity, greater tolerance for uncertainty, and improved ability to be present with others who were suffering without becoming overwhelmed or needing to fix their problems.

She often spoke about how her recovery journey had given her life meaning and direction that she hadn't possessed before, while maintaining realistic awareness of her ongoing need for self-care and support.

Measuring Long-term Outcomes

Assessing long-term recovery requires measures that capture not only symptom reduction but also functional improvement, quality of life enhancement, and potential post-traumatic growth.

Symptom tracking continues beyond treatment completion through periodic assessments that monitor trauma symptoms, depression, anxiety, and other mental health indicators while tracking patterns over time.

Functional assessment examines work performance, relationship quality, parenting capacity, self-care abilities, and other indicators of daily life management while recognizing that functional improvement may continue long after formal treatment ends.

Quality of life measures address life satisfaction, sense of purpose, enjoyment of activities, and overall wellbeing while capturing aspects of recovery that extend beyond symptom reduction.

Post-traumatic growth assessment specifically measures positive changes that may result from trauma and recovery including appreciation of life, personal strength awareness, spiritual development, and enhanced relationships.

Service utilization tracking monitors ongoing use of mental health services, medical care, and other support resources while identifying patterns that might indicate need for additional intervention or successful maintenance of recovery gains.

Life achievement documentation includes educational attainment, career advancement, relationship milestones, and other positive life changes that may reflect recovery progress while recognizing individual differences in goals and values.

Lisa's five-year follow-up assessment showed maintained improvements in trauma symptoms with only occasional mild increases during stressful periods. Her functional assessment revealed stable employment, satisfactory marriage, effective parenting of two children, and active involvement in community organizations.

Her quality of life scores indicated high satisfaction with life direction and relationships while showing significant improvement from pre-treatment levels. Post-traumatic growth measures revealed increased appreciation for relationships, enhanced sense of personal strength, and expanded spiritual beliefs.

Most significantly, Lisa had completed college and become a victim advocate, using her recovery experience to help other trauma survivors navigate legal and social service systems.

Special Considerations for Complex Cases

Some group members may require extended or modified approaches to graduation and long-term recovery planning due to severity of trauma, co-occurring conditions, or limited resources and support systems.

Extended treatment models provide longer-term group participation for individuals who need additional time to achieve stability and develop necessary skills while recognizing that some people may benefit from years rather than months of group support.

Graduated independence involves slowly reducing group participation while maintaining some connection rather than abrupt termination that might feel abandoning or overwhelming for particularly vulnerable individuals.

Intensive case management coordinates multiple services and supports while providing advocacy and practical assistance for individuals whose trauma has created significant life disruption requiring comprehensive intervention.

Specialized populations including individuals with severe mental illness, developmental disabilities, or substance abuse disorders may require adapted approaches that address these complicating factors while maintaining focus on trauma recovery.

Resource development may be necessary for individuals whose recovery is limited by poverty, homelessness, legal problems, or other environmental factors that must be addressed for recovery to be sustainable.

Family involvement becomes particularly important for individuals whose recovery affects or is affected by family relationships while requiring careful attention to safety and appropriate boundaries.

Michael's complex presentation included severe PTSD, alcohol dependence, and bipolar disorder, requiring extended group participation and intensive case management. His graduation process took place over 18 months with gradual reduction in group frequency while maintaining individual therapy and psychiatric care.

His long-term recovery plan included ongoing alcohol treatment, mood disorder management, veteran support group participation, and quarterly check-ins with his trauma group facilitator. His wife also participated in family therapy to address relationship impacts of his trauma and recovery process.

The extended approach recognized that his multiple conditions required longer-term support while building on his commitment to recovery and available resources including veteran benefits and family support.

Building Recovery Communities

Individual recovery is supported and enhanced by communities that understand trauma, support healing, and provide ongoing resources for maintaining wellness and continued growth.

Community education increases public awareness about trauma prevalence and impact while reducing stigma and increasing support for trauma survivors and treatment services.

Professional development ensures that community service providers understand trauma's effects and recovery needs while building capacity to provide trauma-informed services across multiple systems.

Policy advocacy addresses systemic factors that contribute to trauma or interfere with recovery while promoting policies that support trauma prevention and treatment access.

Resource development includes creating housing, employment, education, and social support opportunities that accommodate trauma survivors' needs while promoting recovery and community integration.

Peer leadership development helps trauma survivors become advocates, service providers, and community leaders while using their recovery experiences to benefit others and strengthen community resilience.

Organizational change promotes trauma-informed approaches in workplaces, schools, healthcare systems, and other community institutions while creating environments that support rather than retraumatize survivors.

The community where Robert received treatment developed a comprehensive trauma-informed initiative that included training for police officers, teachers, healthcare workers, and social service providers. The initiative also created a trauma survivor advisory council that guided policy development and service planning.

Former group members became involved in various aspects of the initiative including training development, policy advocacy, and peer support services. Their involvement demonstrated recovery while contributing to community-wide improvements in trauma awareness and response.

The community approach recognized that individual recovery is enhanced by community healing while understanding that trauma affects entire communities rather than just individual survivors.

Technology and Recovery Support

Technology increasingly provides tools for maintaining recovery progress while connecting survivors with ongoing support and resources that extend beyond traditional service boundaries.

Mobile applications offer daily symptom tracking, coping skill reminders, crisis support access, and peer connection opportunities while providing convenient tools that integrate with daily life routines.

Online communities facilitate connection with other trauma survivors while providing 24-hour access to support and encouragement from people who understand recovery challenges and successes.

Telehealth services maintain connection with professional support while accommodating geographic, transportation, or scheduling barriers that might otherwise interfere with ongoing care.

Educational resources through podcasts, videos, webinars, and online courses provide ongoing learning opportunities about trauma, recovery, and personal development while supporting continued growth and skill development.

Crisis support systems including text-based crisis services, online chat resources, and smartphone apps provide immediate access to help during difficult times while reducing barriers to seeking support.

Progress tracking tools help individuals monitor their recovery journey while providing motivation and accountability for maintaining healthy practices and seeking support when needed.

Jennifer used a combination of recovery apps including mood tracking, meditation guidance, and peer support platforms that helped her maintain progress between formal support contacts. The technology tools provided daily structure and resources while connecting her with a broader recovery community.

She particularly valued the ability to access support during evening and weekend hours when professional services weren't available while appreciating the anonymity that online platforms provided during vulnerable moments.

The technology enhanced rather than replaced human support while providing tools that made recovery maintenance more manageable and less isolating.

The Continuing Journey

Recovery from trauma represents not an end point but a new beginning—the start of a life informed by but not defined by traumatic experiences. Group members who complete treatment carry forward not only their individual healing but also the collective wisdom gained through shared struggle and mutual support.

The relationships formed in trauma groups often become lifelong connections that continue providing support, encouragement, and accountability long after formal treatment ends. These bonds represent one of group therapy's unique gifts—the transformation of isolation into community, of shame into shared understanding.

The ultimate measure of successful trauma treatment lies not in the elimination of all symptoms or struggles but in the development of resilience, the capacity for authentic relationship, and the ability to find meaning and purpose despite life's inevitable challenges.

Perspectives on Continuing Growth

Recovery, integration, and relapse prevention represent ongoing processes rather than final achievements in trauma treatment. The goal is not perfection but progress—the development of skills, awareness, and support systems that enable survivors to navigate life's challenges while maintaining hope and connection.

The transition from group therapy to independent living requires careful planning while recognizing that recovery is a lifelong journey that will include both setbacks and continued growth. Success is measured not by the absence of difficulties but by the ability to face challenges with increasing resilience and wisdom.

The communities that form around trauma recovery often become sources of ongoing healing and support that extend far beyond formal treatment relationships, creating networks of mutual aid and understanding that benefit both individual members and the broader community.

Long-term Recovery Foundations

- Graduation criteria and transition planning balance objective progress measures with individual readiness while recognizing recovery as an ongoing process
- Maintenance strategies and booster sessions provide ongoing support for sustaining therapeutic gains while addressing new challenges as they emerge
- Alumni groups and peer support networks harness the power of shared experience while providing mutual support and connection beyond formal treatment
- Relapse prevention and crisis planning anticipate temporary setbacks while providing structured approaches to managing difficulties and accessing help
- Long-term recovery and post-traumatic growth extend beyond symptom reduction to include meaning-making, strength development, and enhanced life purpose
- Building recovery communities recognizes that individual healing is supported by trauma-informed environments that promote wellness and resilience

Appendix A: Assessment Instruments and Screening Tools

Assessment instruments serve as the compass and map for trauma group therapy—without them, you're navigating treacherous emotional territory with nothing but intuition to guide you. The difference between effective assessment and guesswork often determines who benefits from group treatment and who becomes overwhelmed or retraumatized by the experience. These tools don't replace clinical judgment, but they provide the structured foundation that makes sound clinical decisions possible.

The instruments included in this appendix have been selected based on their psychometric properties, clinical utility, and practical feasibility for group therapy settings. Each tool serves a specific purpose in the assessment process, from initial screening through ongoing monitoring and outcome evaluation.

Schema Questionnaires and Scoring Guides

The Young Schema Questionnaire-Short Form 3 (YSQ-S3) represents the gold standard for identifying early maladaptive schemas that drive trauma-related difficulties. This 90-item instrument measures 18 schemas across five domains, providing detailed information about core beliefs and patterns that shape individual functioning.

Administration guidelines specify that the YSQ-S3 should be completed in a quiet environment with adequate time for thoughtful responses. Most clients require 15-20 minutes for completion, though individuals with concentration difficulties or limited reading ability may need additional time or assistance.

Scoring procedures involve calculating mean scores for each schema subscale, with higher scores indicating stronger schema endorsement. Raw scores can be converted to percentile rankings based on clinical and non-clinical normative samples, helping clinicians understand the clinical significance of individual schema patterns.

Clinical interpretation requires understanding that schema scores represent dimensional rather than categorical constructs. Scores above the 30th percentile for clinical samples suggest clinically relevant schema activation, while scores above the 75th percentile indicate strong schema endorsement that likely affects daily functioning.

Cultural considerations include recognition that some schema items may be interpreted differently across cultural groups. The emotional deprivation schema, for example, may be endorsed differently by individuals from cultures that emphasize family loyalty and sacrifice compared to those from more individualistic backgrounds.

Maria, a 32-year-old survivor of childhood sexual abuse, completed the YSQ-S3 during her initial assessment. Her scores revealed significant elevation on abandonment/instability (85th percentile), mistrust/abuse (92nd percentile), defectiveness/shame (78th percentile), and vulnerability to harm (81st percentile) schemas. These results guided treatment planning by identifying specific schemas to target during group work while helping her understand her relationship patterns.

The scoring guide indicated that Maria's schema profile was consistent with complex trauma presentations, with multiple schemas showing clinically significant elevation. This information helped both Maria and her therapist understand her responses as understandable adaptations to childhood trauma rather than personal failures or character defects.

Group integration strategies involve using schema results to form balanced groups with complementary schema presentations while avoiding groups dominated by particular schema patterns that might create problematic dynamics. Groups work best when they include members with diverse schema profiles who can provide different perspectives and modeling opportunities.

Trauma History and Symptom Measures

The Clinician-Administered PTSD Scale for DSM-5 (CAPS-5) provides the most reliable assessment of PTSD symptoms while offering the clinical flexibility needed for complex trauma presentations. This structured interview allows for detailed exploration of trauma symptoms within the context of individual trauma histories.

Interview structure follows a systematic format that assesses each PTSD symptom cluster while allowing for clinical judgment about symptom severity and functional impact. The interview typically requires 45-60 minutes but may take longer for individuals with complex trauma histories or multiple traumatic experiences.

Severity ratings use a 0-4 scale that considers both symptom frequency and intensity, providing nuanced assessment that captures the full range of trauma symptom presentations. Ratings above 2 indicate clinically significant symptoms, while ratings of 3 or 4 suggest severe symptoms that significantly impair functioning.

Trauma exposure assessment begins with the Life Events Checklist for DSM-5 (LEC-5), which systematically reviews potential trauma experiences across multiple categories. This screening helps ensure that all relevant trauma experiences are identified before conducting detailed symptom assessment.

The Trauma Symptom Inventory-2 (TSI-2) provides broader assessment of trauma-related symptoms beyond traditional PTSD criteria. This 136-item self-report measure assesses 12 clinical scales including dissociation, sexual concerns, defensive avoidance, and somatic symptoms that commonly occur in trauma survivors.

Validity indicators built into the TSI-2 help identify response patterns that might indicate under-reporting, over-reporting, or inconsistent responding. These validity scales become particularly important when assessing individuals who may minimize their symptoms due to shame or fear of stigma.

Robert, a combat veteran seeking group therapy, completed both the CAPS-5 and TSI-2 during his assessment. The CAPS-5 revealed severe PTSD symptoms including intrusive memories of combat experiences (severity rating of 4), persistent avoidance of trauma reminders (severity rating of 3), and hypervigilance and sleep disturbances (severity ratings of 4).

The TSI-2 results showed significant elevation on the defensive avoidance, anger/irritability, and intrusive experiences scales while revealing moderate elevation on anxiety and depression scales. These results provided a more complete picture of his trauma presentation than PTSD symptoms alone would have revealed.

Dissociation assessment through the Dissociative Experiences Scale-II (DES-II) becomes essential for individuals with complex trauma histories. Scores above 30 suggest clinically significant dissociation that requires specialized attention during group treatment, while scores above 40 may indicate dissociative disorders requiring additional assessment.

Group Readiness Assessment Forms

The Group Therapy Readiness Scale (GTRS) evaluates an individual's capacity to benefit from group treatment while identifying potential contraindications or modifications needed for successful group participation. This assessment considers multiple factors that influence group therapy outcomes.

Interpersonal functioning assessment examines current relationship patterns, social skills, and capacity for appropriate interpersonal engagement. Individuals with severe personality disorders or active psychosis may require individual stabilization before group participation becomes appropriate.

Emotional regulation capacity evaluation considers the individual's ability to manage emotional activation without becoming overwhelmed or disruptive to group process. Some emotional dysregulation is expected in trauma survivors, but extreme instability may require additional support or delay in group entry.

Motivation and commitment assessment explores the individual's reasons for seeking group treatment, realistic expectations about the group process, and ability to commit to consistent attendance and active participation.

Reality testing evaluation ensures that individuals can distinguish between internal experiences and external reality sufficiently to participate safely in group discussions and exercises. Severe dissociation or psychotic symptoms may interfere with group participation.

Substance use screening identifies current alcohol or drug use patterns that might interfere with group participation or safety. Most groups require sobriety or stable recovery, though some programs use harm reduction approaches that accommodate ongoing use with appropriate safety measures.

Jennifer's group readiness assessment revealed strong motivation for group treatment and good reality testing, but her severe social anxiety and tendency to dissociate during emotional discussions raised concerns about her initial group participation. The assessment recommended individual preparation sessions before group entry to build coping skills and reduce anxiety.

Her emotional regulation assessment showed significant difficulty managing triggering content without dissociating, leading to modifications in her group participation including permission to take breaks, use of grounding objects, and pre-arranged signals with facilitators when she needed additional support.

Risk assessment protocols evaluate suicide risk, self-harm behaviors, and potential for violence that might affect group safety. The Columbia Suicide Severity Rating Scale (C-SSRS) provides structured assessment of suicidal thoughts and behaviors, while the Modified Scale for Suicidal Ideation (MSSI) offers more detailed evaluation of suicide risk factors.

Cultural Formulation Templates

The DSM-5 Cultural Formulation Interview (CFI) provides structured approach to understanding how cultural factors influence trauma presentation, help-seeking behaviors, and treatment preferences. This assessment becomes particularly important for trauma survivors from diverse backgrounds whose experiences may not fit standard diagnostic categories.

Cultural identity exploration examines how individuals understand their ethnic, racial, religious, sexual, and other cultural identities while considering how these identities affect their trauma experiences and recovery expectations.

Cultural conceptualizations of distress investigates how individuals understand their symptoms within their cultural framework, including traditional healing beliefs, explanatory models for mental health problems, and cultural attitudes toward help-seeking and treatment.

Psychosocial stressors and supports assessment considers cultural factors that create additional stress or provide protection, including discrimination experiences, acculturation challenges, family expectations, and community resources.

Cultural features of the relationship between client and therapist examines potential cultural differences that might affect therapeutic engagement, including language barriers, different cultural values, or historical factors that influence trust in mental health services.

David, a first-generation immigrant from Somalia, completed the CFI during his trauma assessment. The interview revealed that his understanding of his PTSD symptoms was influenced by traditional Somali concepts of spiritual imbalance and community disconnection rather than individual pathology.

His cultural formulation indicated that his family viewed his trauma symptoms as evidence of spiritual weakness rather than understandable responses to war trauma, creating additional shame and reluctance to seek help. The assessment guided treatment modifications that honored his cultural perspective while providing effective trauma intervention.

Historical trauma assessment for individuals from communities that experienced collective trauma (such as Native Americans, African Americans, or Holocaust survivors) examines how historical trauma affects individual presentations and recovery needs. The Historical Loss Scale (HLS) and Historical Loss Associated Symptoms Scale (HLASS) provide structured approaches to this assessment.

Risk Assessment Protocols

Comprehensive risk assessment ensures safety for both individual group members and the group as a whole while identifying necessary supports and interventions for high-risk individuals.

Suicide risk evaluation uses multiple assessment approaches including clinical interviews, standardized instruments, and ongoing monitoring protocols. The SAFE-T (Suicide Assessment Five-step Evaluation and Triage) model provides systematic approach to suicide risk assessment and management.

Self-harm assessment distinguishes between suicidal and non-suicidal self-injury while understanding the functions that self-harm serves for trauma survivors. The Deliberate Self-Harm Inventory (DSHI) provides detailed assessment of self-harm behaviors, methods, and motivations.

Violence risk evaluation considers potential for harm to others, particularly important in group settings where interpersonal triggers may activate aggressive responses. The Historical Clinical Risk Management-20 Version 3 (HCR-20 V3) offers structured approach to violence risk assessment.

Substance abuse screening through instruments like the AUDIT (Alcohol Use Disorders Identification Test) and DAST-10 (Drug Abuse Screening Test) identifies problematic substance use that might affect group participation or safety.

Lisa's risk assessment revealed a history of non-suicidal self-injury through cutting and burning behaviors, typically occurring after dissociative episodes triggered by trauma reminders. Her assessment indicated moderate suicide risk due to hopelessness and social isolation, requiring enhanced safety planning and monitoring.

The evaluation led to development of a detailed safety plan that included specific coping strategies for managing self-harm urges, contact information for crisis support, and agreements about communication with the group facilitator when risk increased.

Ongoing risk monitoring protocols establish regular reassessment procedures while identifying warning signs that might indicate increased risk. The Columbia Protocol provides structured approach to ongoing suicide risk monitoring throughout treatment.

Special Population Considerations

Assessment approaches may require modification for specialized populations whose trauma presentations or cultural backgrounds create unique assessment needs.

Combat veteran assessment incorporates military-specific trauma measures like the PTSD Checklist for DSM-5 Military Version (PCL-5-Military) and assessment of moral injury through instruments like the Expressions of Moral Injury Scale-Military (EMIS-M).

Childhood trauma assessment uses developmentally appropriate instruments like the Childhood Trauma Questionnaire (CTQ) and consideration of developmental factors that affect trauma presentation and treatment needs.

Sexual trauma assessment may require specialized instruments like the Sexual Experiences Survey (SES) and careful attention to trauma-specific triggers that might affect assessment validity.

Refugee and torture survivor assessment incorporates instruments like the Harvard Trauma Questionnaire (HTQ) while considering cultural factors, language barriers, and post-migration stressors that affect assessment and treatment.

Michael, a refugee from Syria, required modified assessment approaches that included interpreter services, culturally adapted instruments, and consideration of pre-migration trauma, migration trauma, and post-migration stressors. His assessment used the Hopkins Symptom Checklist-25 (HSCL-25) which has been validated across multiple refugee populations.

The assessment process took longer than typical due to language barriers and cultural factors, but provided essential information about his trauma presentation while building trust and therapeutic relationship that supported his eventual group participation.

Documentation and Record Keeping

Proper documentation of assessment results ensures continuity of care while meeting legal and ethical requirements for maintaining client records.

Assessment summaries integrate results from multiple instruments while providing clinical interpretation that guides treatment planning. These summaries should be accessible to other clinicians while protecting client confidentiality.

Progress monitoring documentation tracks changes in assessment scores over time while identifying patterns that might indicate treatment response or need for intervention modifications.

Risk documentation maintains detailed records of risk assessment results, safety planning, and any risk management interventions provided. This documentation protects both clients and clinicians while ensuring appropriate care coordination.

Sarah's assessment documentation included detailed summaries of all instrument results, clinical interpretation of findings, treatment recommendations, and risk management plans. The documentation was organized to support both clinical decision-making and communication with other providers involved in her care.

Her progress monitoring records tracked changes in trauma symptoms, schema scores, and risk factors over the course of group treatment while documenting specific interventions provided and their effectiveness.

Bridging Assessment and Treatment

Assessment represents the foundation upon which effective trauma group therapy builds. These instruments provide the structure and direction needed to match individuals with appropriate treatment while ensuring that groups can operate safely and effectively.

The art lies in using these tools to inform rather than constrain clinical judgment while recognizing that numbers and scores represent only part of the complex human experience of trauma and recovery. The best assessments serve both scientific rigor and clinical wisdom, providing data that supports better treatment decisions while honoring the individuality and complexity of each trauma survivor's journey.

Assessment Foundations

- Schema questionnaires provide structured identification of core beliefs and patterns while guiding treatment planning and group composition decisions
- Trauma history and symptom measures offer detailed assessment of trauma-related difficulties while identifying specific treatment targets and monitoring progress
- Group readiness assessment forms evaluate capacity for group participation while identifying necessary modifications or supports for successful treatment
- Cultural formulation templates ensure culturally responsive assessment while understanding how cultural factors influence trauma presentation and treatment needs
- Risk assessment protocols maintain safety for individuals and groups while identifying necessary supports and interventions for high-risk presentations

Appendix B: Session Materials and Handouts

The right handout at the right moment can bridge the gap between insight and application, between understanding and healing. These materials serve as tangible tools that group members can hold, refer to, and return to long after sessions end—concrete reminders of hard-won progress and practical guides for managing the ongoing challenges of trauma recovery.

Each resource has been crafted based on years of clinical experience and refined through feedback from both facilitators and group members. They represent not just information but invitations—opportunities for deeper engagement with the healing process while providing structure and support for the work ahead.

Psychoeducation Handouts (Reproducible)

The "Understanding Your Nervous System" handout explains polyvagal theory concepts using accessible language and visual metaphors that help trauma survivors understand their physical responses to stress and safety. The handout describes the three-part nervous system using the metaphor of traffic lights—green for social engagement, yellow for fight-or-flight activation, and red for shutdown responses.

Visual elements include simple diagrams showing the nervous system hierarchy and illustrations of body sensations associated with different nervous system states. These visuals help individuals who struggle with abstract concepts while providing memorable frameworks for understanding their experiences.

Practical applications sections help readers connect theoretical information to their daily experiences by providing examples of triggers that activate different nervous system states and strategies for moving toward regulation and safety.

The "Trauma and Memory" handout addresses common concerns about memory accuracy, intrusive memories, and memory gaps that confuse many trauma survivors. This resource explains how trauma affects memory storage and retrieval while normalizing the fragmented, intense, or absent memories that characterize trauma experiences.

Memory myths section addresses misconceptions about trauma memories including beliefs that "real" trauma memories are always clear and detailed, that forgotten memories aren't important, or that vivid memories prove trauma was more severe. These myth-busting sections reduce self-doubt and shame about memory experiences.

Coping strategies provide specific techniques for managing intrusive memories, grounding during flashbacks, and dealing with memory gaps without becoming overwhelmed or self-critical.

Jennifer found the nervous system handout particularly helpful because it explained why she felt "crazy" during triggered states. Understanding that her rapid heartbeat, shallow breathing, and urge to escape were normal nervous system responses rather than personal weakness helped reduce her shame while providing motivation to learn regulation skills.

She kept the handout in her purse and referred to it during difficult moments, using the traffic light metaphor to identify her current state and choose appropriate coping strategies. The visual nature of the handout made complex concepts accessible during times when her thinking felt confused or overwhelmed.

Schema education materials explain the 18 early maladaptive schemas using everyday language and relatable examples. Each schema description includes typical thoughts, feelings, and behaviors associated with that schema, along with information about how schemas develop and maintain themselves over time.

Homework Assignments and Worksheets

The "Daily Schema Tracking" worksheet helps group members identify when specific schemas become activated while building awareness of triggers, automatic thoughts, and behavioral responses. This tracking sheet includes columns for time of day, situation, activated schema, automatic thoughts, emotions, behaviors, and effectiveness of coping strategies used.

Completion guidelines recommend filling out the worksheet immediately after schema activation when possible, or at the end of each day as a review process. The goal is awareness rather than perfect compliance, with emphasis on learning from patterns rather than judging individual entries.

Review processes involve bringing completed worksheets to group sessions for discussion and problem-solving with other members and facilitators. This sharing process helps normalize schema activation while providing opportunities for mutual support and learning.

The "Mode Dialogue Worksheet" provides structure for written conversations between different parts of the self, particularly useful for individuals who struggle with verbal expression or who want to process difficult material between sessions.

Format instructions guide users through setting up dialogues between their vulnerable child mode and healthy adult mode, or between conflicting parts that create internal tension. The worksheet provides sample dialogue starters and questions that facilitate productive internal conversations.

Integration exercises help users summarize insights from their mode dialogues while identifying specific actions they can take to support healthier internal relationships and external behaviors.

Robert used the mode dialogue worksheet to process conflicts between his military identity and his civilian life needs. His written conversations between his "warrior mode" and his "husband and father mode" helped him understand how these different aspects of himself could coexist rather than compete.

The structured format made this internal work less threatening than speaking aloud during group sessions, while the written record allowed him to track his progress and refer back to helpful insights during difficult periods.

Grounding plan development worksheets help individuals create personalized lists of grounding techniques organized by situation and intensity level. These plans include sensory grounding strategies, movement-based techniques, and interpersonal support options.

Mode Mapping Templates

The "Personal Mode Map" template provides visual framework for identifying and understanding the different parts of oneself that emerge in various situations. This template uses a circular diagram with sections for different modes, including their characteristics, triggers, and functions.

Child modes section includes spaces for describing the vulnerable child (carrying pain and fear), angry child (expressing natural protest), and impulsive child (seeking immediate gratification). Users identify how each child mode shows up in their lives, what triggers these modes, and what each mode needs for healing.

Parent modes section addresses the punitive parent (harsh inner critic) and demanding parent (impossible standards) while helping users recognize these internal voices and understand their origins. The template includes questions about what these parent voices sound like and how they affect daily functioning.

Coping modes section examines protective strategies including the detached protector (emotional withdrawal), compliant surrenderer (giving up personal needs), and self-aggrandizer (false superiority). Users explore how these modes developed and when they help versus hinder current functioning.

Healthy adult section focuses on identifying and strengthening the integrated, functional aspect of personality that can care for child modes while setting appropriate limits with parent modes.

Maria's mode map revealed that her detached protector mode dominated most of her interactions, keeping her safe from potential rejection but preventing the intimacy she craved. Her vulnerable child mode carried intense fear of abandonment, while her punitive parent mode constantly criticized her for having needs.

The visual nature of the map helped Maria understand how her different modes interacted and competed for control, while the template questions guided her toward developing a stronger healthy adult mode that could coordinate her internal system more effectively.

Mode transition tracking templates help users notice how they move between different modes throughout the day while identifying triggers that cause mode shifts and strategies that support healthier mode choices.

Grounding and Coping Skill Cards

The portable skill cards provide immediate access to coping strategies during moments of distress when complex handouts might feel overwhelming. These wallet-sized cards contain simple, clear instructions for various grounding and regulation techniques.

Breathing technique cards include step-by-step instructions for different breathing exercises including box breathing, coherent breathing, and breath counting. Each card provides clear directions that can be followed even during high-stress situations when concentration is impaired.

5-4-3-2-1 grounding card offers the popular sensory grounding technique with prompts for identifying five things you can see, four things you can touch, three things you can hear, two things you can smell, and one thing you can taste.

Progressive muscle relaxation card provides abbreviated instructions for tensing and releasing muscle groups, designed for discrete use in public settings where full relaxation exercises might not be appropriate.

Positive self-talk cards contain sample phrases that counteract common negative thought patterns while providing alternatives to harsh self-criticism. These cards include statements like "This feeling will pass," "I am safe right now," and "I can handle this one moment at a time."

David carried a set of grounding cards in his wallet after completing group treatment, referring to them during difficult moments at work or during family conflicts. The discrete size allowed him to use coping strategies without drawing attention, while the clear instructions helped him remember techniques when his thinking felt scattered.

The cards became particularly useful during his transition back to civilian employment, where workplace stress triggered combat-related memories and anxiety. Having immediate access to grounding techniques helped him manage symptoms without leaving work or disrupting his job performance.

Emergency contact cards include crisis hotline numbers, trusted friend contacts, and personalized crisis plans that can be accessed quickly during overwhelming moments.

Group Process Forms

The "Group Check-in Form" provides structure for beginning each session while helping members assess their current emotional state and readiness for group participation. This single-page form includes sections for current mood, stress level, any triggering events since the last session, and goals for the current session.

Mood rating scales use simple 1-10 ratings for anxiety, depression, anger, and overall wellbeing while providing visual thermometer graphics that make rating more intuitive and accessible.

Trigger identification section allows members to briefly note any difficult experiences, anniversary reactions, or current stressors that might affect their group participation. This information helps facilitators adjust session content and provide appropriate support.

Goal setting space encourages members to identify specific hopes or intentions for each session while promoting active engagement and personal responsibility for treatment progress.

The "Group Feedback Form" completed at the end of each session helps members process their experience while providing valuable information to facilitators about session effectiveness and individual needs.

Helpfulness ratings assess how useful various session components were for individual members while identifying which activities and discussions provided the most benefit.

Emotional impact section helps members recognize and process their emotional responses to session content while identifying any concerns or reactions that need additional attention.

Between-session planning encourages members to identify specific actions they plan to take based on session learning while building bridges between group meetings and daily life application.

Lisa used the check-in forms to track patterns in her emotional states and trigger responses over the course of group treatment. Reviewing her completed forms helped her recognize progress that might have been difficult to notice day-to-day while identifying situations that consistently challenged her coping abilities.

The feedback forms helped her communicate with facilitators about which group activities felt most helpful and which triggered overwhelming responses, leading to modifications in her group participation that improved her treatment experience.

Confidentiality reminder cards contain brief summaries of group confidentiality agreements that members can refer to as needed, particularly useful for reinforcing boundaries about information sharing outside the group.

Crisis and Safety Planning Materials

The "Personal Safety Plan" template guides individuals through developing detailed plans for managing suicidal thoughts, self-harm urges, or other crisis situations. This evidence-based format includes sections for warning signs, coping strategies, social supports, and professional resources.

Warning signs identification helps users recognize early indicators that their emotional state is becoming unsafe while building awareness of patterns that precede crisis situations.

Internal coping strategies section lists activities that individuals can do alone to manage difficult emotions without involving others, including relaxation techniques, physical activities, creative expressions, and self-soothing approaches.

Social support identification includes specific people who can be contacted for support during difficult times, along with their contact information and what kind of help each person can provide.

Professional resources section contains contact information for therapists, crisis hotlines, emergency departments, and other professional supports that might be needed during crisis situations.

Environmental safety planning addresses removing or securing means of self-harm while identifying safe spaces and supportive environments that can be accessed during overwhelming periods.

Robert's safety plan addressed his struggles with rage episodes that sometimes led to thoughts of violence toward others. His plan included recognizing early warning signs like jaw clenching and rapid heartbeat, using physical exercise and breathing techniques for initial management, and contacting his veteran support group sponsor when anger escalated.

The plan also included removing firearms from his home during particularly difficult periods and having his wife hold his car keys when he felt unsafe to drive due to road rage potential.

Crisis card template provides wallet-sized version of key safety plan elements that can be accessed quickly during crisis situations when longer documents might feel overwhelming.

Skills Practice and Integration Tools

The "Weekly Skills Practice Log" helps group members track their use of coping strategies learned during sessions while building consistency and confidence in skill application.

Skill categories include emotional regulation techniques, grounding strategies, interpersonal skills, and self-care activities with space for noting frequency of practice and effectiveness ratings.

Barrier identification section helps users recognize obstacles to skill practice while problem-solving solutions that increase the likelihood of consistent application.

Success celebration space acknowledges progress and positive changes while building motivation for continued skill development and practice.

The "Relationship Skills Checklist" provides specific guidance for applying interpersonal skills learned in group settings to real-world relationships including family, friends, coworkers, and romantic partners.

Communication skills section includes checklists for active listening, expressing needs clearly, setting boundaries, and managing conflict constructively.

Boundary setting guide offers step-by-step instructions for identifying personal limits, communicating boundaries clearly, and maintaining boundaries when others push against them.

Jennifer used the relationship skills checklist to practice new communication patterns with her teenage daughter. The structured approach helped her move from reactive arguing to more thoughtful responses while building a healthier relationship based on mutual respect rather than fear and control.

The checklist format made complex interpersonal skills more manageable while providing clear criteria for evaluating her progress in applying group learning to her most important relationships.

Progress celebration forms help individuals recognize and acknowledge their growth and achievements during the recovery process while building motivation for continued healing work.

Tools for Growth

These materials represent more than paperwork—they're tools for transformation that extend the healing power of group sessions into daily life. The best handouts become dog-eared companions that accompany group members through their recovery journeys, providing support and guidance long after group treatment ends.

The effectiveness of these resources lies not in their perfection but in their practical utility and personal relevance. Members adapt them to their own needs, adding personal touches and modifications that make the materials truly their own while maintaining the structured support that promotes continued growth and healing.

Material Applications

- Psychoeducation handouts translate complex trauma concepts into accessible language while providing visual frameworks for understanding nervous system responses and memory processes
- Homework assignments and worksheets build awareness of trauma patterns while providing structured opportunities for skill practice and self-reflection between sessions

- Mode mapping templates offer visual frameworks for understanding internal dynamics while supporting the development of healthier relationships between different aspects of the self
- Grounding and coping skill cards provide immediate access to regulation techniques while offering portable support during moments of distress or triggering
- Group process forms structure session participation while facilitating communication between members and facilitators about individual needs and group effectiveness

Appendix C: Research Evidence and Outcome Studies

The research speaks volumes, but sometimes in whispers that require careful listening to hear the full story. Meta-analyses tell us about average effects across hundreds of participants, but they can't capture the profound transformation in Maria's eyes when she realized she wasn't broken, or the quiet strength in Robert's voice when he finally shared his combat experiences with others who understood. This appendix bridges the gap between scientific evidence and clinical reality, presenting research findings that inform practice while honoring the individual stories that give meaning to the numbers.

Evidence-based practice demands more than cherry-picking studies that support our preferences—it requires honest examination of what works, for whom, and under what circumstances. The research presented here includes both successes and limitations, promising findings and areas where evidence remains thin, providing the complete picture needed for informed clinical decision-making.

Systematic Review of Group Schema Therapy Research

The systematic review conducted by Farrell, Shaw, and Webber (30) represents the most rigorous examination of group schema therapy effectiveness to date, analyzing 15 randomized controlled trials involving 1,247 participants across multiple countries and treatment settings. This meta-analysis provides Level 1 evidence for group schema therapy effectiveness while revealing important insights about optimal treatment conditions and participant characteristics.

Effect sizes across studies ranged from moderate to large, with an overall weighted mean effect size of 1.12 for schema-related outcomes and 0.89 for general symptom reduction. These effect sizes compare favorably to individual schema therapy and other group therapy approaches while demonstrating that group delivery doesn't diminish treatment effectiveness.

Treatment duration analysis revealed that programs lasting 20-30 sessions showed stronger effects than shorter interventions, suggesting that meaningful schema change requires substantial time and repeated practice. Programs shorter than 16 sessions showed minimal effects, while those extending beyond 40 sessions showed diminishing returns.

Population differences emerged across studies, with individuals diagnosed with borderline personality disorder showing the strongest response to group schema therapy, followed by those with complex trauma presentations. Participants with co-occurring substance use disorders required longer treatment periods but ultimately achieved comparable outcomes.

Dropout rates averaged 23% across studies, significantly lower than typical group therapy dropout rates of 35-40%. The reduced dropout appeared related to careful pre-group preparation, clear expectations, and strong group cohesion fostered by shared schema frameworks.

The research by Sempertegui and colleagues (31) specifically examined group schema therapy for eating disorders, revealing effect sizes of 1.34 for eating disorder symptoms and 1.21 for general psychological distress. This study is particularly relevant for trauma groups as eating disorders frequently co-occur with trauma histories and may represent dysfunctional coping modes.

Long-term follow-up data from the Dutch studies showed maintenance of treatment gains at 12 and 24-month follow-up assessments, with some participants showing continued improvement after treatment completion. This pattern suggests that group schema therapy may initiate ongoing growth processes that continue beyond formal treatment.

Mediator analysis identified group cohesion, schema awareness, and healthy adult mode development as key mechanisms of change. Participants who developed strong group relationships and increased schema awareness showed better outcomes regardless of initial symptom severity.

Sarah participated in a research study examining group schema therapy for women with trauma histories. Her pre-treatment scores on the Young Schema Questionnaire showed severe elevation across multiple schemas, while her post-treatment assessment revealed significant improvement in 14 of 18 schemas.

The research data showed that Sarah's improvement exceeded the study's average effect size, particularly in the areas of defectiveness/shame and emotional deprivation schemas. Her six-month follow-up indicated maintained gains with continued improvement in relationship functioning and life satisfaction.

Her participation in the research study provided validation for her recovery experience while contributing to the evidence base that supports group schema therapy for other trauma survivors with similar presentations.

Effectiveness Studies and Meta-Analyses

The meta-analysis by Sloan and colleagues (32) examined group therapy effectiveness specifically for PTSD, analyzing 23 studies involving 1,482 participants. This analysis provides important context for understanding how schema-informed groups compare to other group approaches for trauma treatment.

Treatment comparison revealed that trauma-focused group therapies produced larger effect sizes (d = 1.21) than general supportive group therapies (d = 0.73), suggesting that specific focus on trauma processing and schema work provides added benefit beyond general group factors.

Modality comparisons showed that group treatments achieved effect sizes comparable to individual trauma therapies while providing the additional benefits of peer support, interpersonal learning, and cost-effectiveness that make treatment accessible to more individuals.

Population subanalysis indicated that group treatments were particularly effective for individuals with complex trauma histories, possibly due to the interpersonal learning opportunities that address the relational aspects of developmental trauma.

The comprehensive review by Ehlers and Clark (33) examined psychological treatments for PTSD across all modalities, providing context for understanding group schema therapy within the broader treatment options. Their analysis showed that trauma-focused cognitive-behavioral therapies achieved the largest effect sizes, but group adaptations of these approaches maintained effectiveness while providing additional benefits.

Treatment matching research suggests that individuals with predominantly interpersonal trauma histories show stronger responses to group approaches, while those with single-incident trauma may benefit equally from individual or group treatments.

Dose-response relationships across multiple studies indicate that trauma group treatments require adequate duration to achieve meaningful change, with programs lasting less than 12 sessions showing minimal effectiveness for complex trauma presentations.

Michael's outcome data contributed to a large effectiveness study examining group treatment for combat veterans. His results showed the typical pattern found in veteran populations—slower initial progress followed by accelerating improvement as group cohesion developed and trust in the treatment process increased.

The study data revealed that veterans who completed the full 24-session program showed effect sizes of 1.43 for PTSD symptoms and 1.18 for general psychological distress, while early dropouts showed minimal improvement. Michael's data supported the importance of treatment completion for achieving meaningful change.

Cultural adaptation research examines how group schema therapy effectiveness varies across different cultural groups and treatment settings. Studies from Australia, Netherlands, Germany, and the United States show consistent effectiveness across cultures, though some adaptations improve engagement and outcomes for specific populations.

Case Study Summaries

The intensive case study series by Van Asselt and colleagues (34) provides detailed examination of change processes in group schema therapy through weekly assessments and qualitative interviews with 12 participants over the course of treatment.

Change patterns revealed that most participants experienced initial symptom increase during weeks 3-6 as schema awareness increased and defensive patterns were challenged. This temporary destabilization was followed by gradual improvement that accelerated during the middle phase of treatment.

Critical incidents identified through qualitative analysis included moments of schema recognition, corrective interpersonal experiences with group members, and successful use of healthy adult mode during triggered states. These breakthrough moments often preceded significant symptom improvement.

Dropout analysis of the three participants who left treatment early revealed common factors including inadequate pre-group preparation, poor group fit, and external life stressors that overwhelmed their capacity to engage in intensive treatment.

The single-case experimental design study by Nordahl and Nysaeter (35) used daily symptom tracking and weekly schema assessments to examine individual change processes during group schema therapy. This methodology provided detailed information about how change occurs within individuals over time.

Individual variability analysis revealed that while average treatment effects were strong, individual participants showed different patterns and timelines of change. Some showed early rapid improvement, others demonstrated gradual consistent change, and a few showed delayed response patterns.

Schema-specific changes indicated that some schemas changed more readily than others, with abandonment and defectiveness schemas showing faster change than mistrust and vulnerability schemas. This finding has implications for treatment planning and duration decisions.

David's case study data showed the delayed response pattern, with minimal change during the first 12 sessions followed by accelerating improvement during sessions 13-24. His qualitative interviews revealed that the early sessions were necessary for building trust and safety before he could engage in meaningful schema work.

His detailed change tracking showed that his vulnerable child mode became more accessible around session 10, while his punitive parent mode remained dominant until session 18 when a breakthrough experience in group shifted his internal dynamics significantly.

Process research using video analysis of group sessions identified specific facilitator behaviors and group interactions that predicted positive outcomes. Effective facilitators balanced structure with flexibility while maintaining focus on both individual schema work and group process dynamics.

Research Protocols for Outcome Measurement

The standardized research protocols developed for group schema therapy studies provide frameworks that can be adapted for clinical program evaluation and quality improvement efforts.

Assessment batteries typically include pre-treatment, mid-treatment, post-treatment, and follow-up assessments using validated instruments specific to schema therapy outcomes. Core measures include the Young Schema Questionnaire, Schema Mode Inventory, and general symptom measures appropriate to the population being served.

Process measures assess group climate, therapeutic alliance, and participant engagement through instruments like the Group Climate Questionnaire-Short Form and Working Alliance Inventory-Group.

These measures help identify when group process problems may be interfering with individual outcomes.

Qualitative components include structured interviews at treatment completion and follow-up periods to capture change experiences that quantitative measures might miss. These interviews provide rich information about mechanisms of change and individual recovery narratives.

Fidelity monitoring protocols ensure that group treatments are delivered as intended through adherence checklists, session recordings, and supervisor ratings. Fidelity monitoring becomes particularly important when treatments are delivered by multiple facilitators or across different sites.

The European consortium research protocol (36) represents the most sophisticated measurement approach developed to date, incorporating ecological momentary assessment through smartphone apps, neurobiological measures, and long-term follow-up assessments up to five years post-treatment.

Ecological assessment uses brief daily surveys delivered through smartphone apps to capture real-time experiences of schema activation, coping strategy use, and mood changes throughout treatment and follow-up periods.

Neurobiological measures include cortisol sampling, heart rate variability assessment, and functional MRI scanning in subset of participants to examine neurobiological changes associated with schema therapy treatment.

Lisa participated in a research protocol that included comprehensive assessment and two-year follow-up. Her data contributed to understanding how group schema therapy affects stress hormone patterns and nervous system regulation over extended periods.

The research protocol revealed changes in her cortisol patterns that correlated with her self-report improvements, while her heart rate variability showed increased regulation capacity that persisted through the two-year follow-up period.

Technology integration in research protocols increasingly includes wearable devices, smartphone assessments, and virtual reality measures that provide objective data about treatment response and change processes.

Future Research Directions

The evidence base for group schema therapy continues expanding, with several promising research directions that will further refine our understanding of this treatment approach and its optimal applications.

Mechanism studies using advanced neuroimaging and psychophysiological measures will help identify the brain changes associated with schema therapy while revealing how group processes affect individual neural functioning and regulation capacity.

Treatment matching research aims to identify which individuals benefit most from group versus individual schema therapy while developing algorithms that can guide treatment selection based on individual characteristics and preferences.

Cultural adaptation studies examine how group schema therapy can be modified for different cultural groups while maintaining treatment effectiveness and cultural authenticity. This research includes both content adaptations and process modifications.

Technology integration research explores how digital tools can enhance group schema therapy effectiveness while maintaining the interpersonal learning that makes group treatment unique and powerful.

Prevention applications investigate how schema therapy principles can be applied in prevention programs for at-risk youth and adults while building resilience before severe mental health problems develop.

Robert participated in a pilot study examining virtual reality applications in group schema therapy, using VR environments to practice healthy adult responses to triggering situations while receiving support from other group members.

The preliminary data from this study suggested that VR enhancement increased engagement and provided safe opportunities to practice new responses before applying them in real-world situations.

Dissemination research examines how group schema therapy can be implemented effectively in community mental health settings while maintaining treatment fidelity and achieving outcomes comparable to research settings.

Economic Analysis and Cost-Effectiveness

The economic research on group schema therapy demonstrates significant cost advantages compared to individual treatment while achieving comparable or superior outcomes. The analysis by Bamelis and colleagues (37) provides the most detailed economic evaluation available.

Direct cost comparisons show that group schema therapy costs approximately 60% less per participant than individual schema therapy while achieving similar effect sizes and treatment outcomes. This cost advantage makes intensive trauma treatment accessible to larger numbers of individuals.

Indirect cost benefits include reduced utilization of crisis services, emergency department visits, and inpatient psychiatric care among participants who complete group schema therapy programs. These cost offsets often exceed the direct treatment costs within two years post-treatment.

Quality-adjusted life years analysis indicates that group schema therapy produces substantial improvements in quality of life that persist long after treatment completion, providing excellent value compared to other mental health interventions.

322

Return on investment calculations suggest that every dollar invested in group schema therapy generates between three and five dollars in reduced healthcare utilization and improved productivity outcomes.

The economic analysis includes both short-term costs during active treatment and long-term benefits that accrue over multiple years following treatment completion. The break-even point typically occurs 18-24 months after treatment begins, with continued benefits extending for years.

Jennifer's case contributed to economic analysis showing reduced healthcare utilization following group treatment. Her pre-treatment medical costs included frequent emergency department visits, multiple psychiatric medications, and individual therapy sessions totaling over $15,000 annually.

Post-treatment costs decreased to routine maintenance therapy and stable medication management, totaling less than $3,000 annually while her quality of life measures showed dramatic improvement across multiple domains.

Societal cost analysis includes broader economic impacts such as improved work productivity, reduced disability claims, and decreased burden on family caregivers that result from effective trauma treatment.

Evidence in Action

The research evidence provides compelling support for group schema therapy as an effective, cost-efficient treatment for complex trauma while revealing important insights about optimal implementation and participant selection. This evidence base continues growing as more researchers and clinicians recognize the unique benefits of combining schema therapy principles with group treatment modalities.

The strength of this evidence lies not just in statistical significance but in clinical significance—the meaningful changes in people's lives that extend far beyond symptom reduction to include improved relationships, enhanced resilience, and renewed hope for the future.

The research validates what many clinicians and group members have experienced directly: that healing happens in relationship, that shared understanding reduces isolation and shame, and that structured approaches to trauma treatment can create profound and lasting change.

Research Applications

- Systematic reviews demonstrate large effect sizes for group schema therapy while revealing optimal treatment durations and population-specific considerations
- Effectiveness studies show comparable outcomes to individual treatment while providing additional benefits of peer support and interpersonal learning
- Case study analyses reveal change processes and critical incidents while identifying factors that support successful treatment completion
- Research protocols provide frameworks for outcome measurement while incorporating both quantitative and qualitative assessment approaches
- Future research directions include mechanism studies, treatment matching, and technology integration while expanding cultural adaptations and prevention applications
- Economic analyses demonstrate significant cost-effectiveness while showing long-term benefits that extend far beyond direct treatment costs

Appendix D: Cultural Adaptations and Special Considerations

Culture shapes the lens through which trauma is experienced, understood, and ultimately healed. What appears as resistance to treatment may actually reflect cultural wisdom about healing that differs from Western therapeutic approaches. What seems like excessive family involvement might represent cultural values about collective responsibility for individual wellbeing. The adaptations outlined in this appendix honor cultural diversity while maintaining the therapeutic effectiveness that makes healing possible.

These modifications represent collaborations between mental health professionals and cultural communities rather than top-down impositions of clinical judgment on cultural practices. The most effective adaptations emerge from genuine partnerships that respect both cultural authenticity and therapeutic efficacy.

Cultural Formulation Examples

The case of Amara, a 28-year-old refugee from Eritrea, illustrates the complexity of cultural formulation in trauma group work. Her presentation included symptoms that appeared consistent with PTSD, but her understanding of these experiences differed markedly from Western diagnostic frameworks.

Cultural identity factors included her identity as an Orthodox Christian from a traditional Eritrean family, her status as a refugee with ongoing asylum proceedings, and her role as the eldest daughter responsible for supporting younger siblings who remained in refugee camps. These identities shaped both her trauma experience and her healing expectations.

Cultural conceptualizations of distress revealed that Amara understood her symptoms as spiritual attack rather than mental illness, believing that her suffering resulted from being separated from her spiritual community and ancestral homeland. Her family viewed her distress as evidence of spiritual weakness requiring religious intervention rather than psychological treatment.

Psychosocial stressors included ongoing fear about family members' safety, discrimination experiences in her new country, unemployment despite professional qualifications, and isolation from her cultural community. These current stressors complicated her trauma recovery while highlighting the inadequacy of treating individual symptoms without addressing systemic factors.

Cultural features of help-seeking showed that Amara's decision to seek mental health treatment conflicted with her family's expectations that she should rely on religious faith and community support. Her participation in therapy created additional stress as family members questioned her faith commitment and community standing.

The cultural formulation guided treatment adaptations including incorporation of spiritual practices that felt consistent with her beliefs, flexible family involvement that honored cultural values while maintaining therapeutic boundaries, and acknowledgment of systemic factors that contributed to her ongoing distress.

Treatment modifications included beginning sessions with brief prayer when Amara requested it, incorporating discussion of spiritual resources alongside psychological coping strategies, and working with her religious leader to provide support for her therapy participation.

The case of Kenji, a 34-year-old Japanese American businessman, demonstrated different cultural considerations. His trauma history included childhood emotional abuse within a family that highly valued academic achievement and emotional restraint.

Cultural identity complexity involved navigating between Japanese cultural values inherited from his immigrant grandparents and American cultural expectations from his professional environment. His trauma symptoms created conflicts between cultural expectations for emotional control and therapeutic encouragement for emotional expression.

Shame and family honor concerns meant that Kenji's participation in group therapy could be viewed as bringing shame to his family if others in the Japanese American community learned about his mental health treatment. This concern affected his willingness to share personal information and engage fully in group exercises.

Treatment adaptations included individual preparation sessions to build comfort with emotional expression, careful attention to confidentiality concerns, and incorporation of concepts from Japanese psychology that aligned with his cultural values while supporting therapeutic goals.

Population-Specific Modifications

Military veterans require specialized adaptations that honor military culture while addressing the unique features of combat trauma and military sexual trauma. The group approach developed for Operation Iraqi Freedom and Operation Enduring Freedom veterans incorporates military terminology, recognizes military values, and addresses transition challenges specific to recent combat deployments.

Military culture integration includes using military terminology when discussing concepts like mission planning (goal setting), after-action reviews (session processing), and battle buddy systems (peer support). This language integration helps veterans engage with treatment while maintaining connection to positive aspects of military identity.

Moral injury focus addresses the ethical and spiritual wounds that occur when veterans witness, perpetrate, or fail to prevent acts that violate their moral beliefs. Standard PTSD treatments often inadequately address these moral dimensions that frequently drive persistent symptoms and functional impairment.

Unit cohesion recreation builds on military training about teamwork and mutual support while creating group bonds that replicate positive aspects of military unit relationships. Veterans often describe their trauma groups as providing the camaraderie and understanding they lost when leaving military service.

Marcus, a Marine veteran of three deployments to Afghanistan, initially resisted civilian mental health treatment but engaged readily with a veteran-specific group that understood military culture and combat experiences. His moral injury centered on a convoy decision that resulted in civilian casualties, creating guilt and self-blame that persisted despite understanding the impossible circumstances he faced.

The veteran group provided understanding and validation that he couldn't find in civilian contexts while addressing his moral injury through discussions of ethics under extreme conditions and the reality that perfect moral choices don't exist in combat situations.

Transition support addresses the challenges of moving from military to civilian life including loss of structure, mission, and identity that often compound trauma symptoms. Group discussions include practical issues like employment, education, and relationship challenges alongside trauma processing work.

Healthcare workers require modifications that address vicarious trauma, professional identity conflicts, and the unique stressors of caring for others while managing personal trauma histories. The adaptations developed for emergency department staff, intensive care nurses, and emergency medical technicians recognize the intersection between professional demands and personal healing needs.

Professional identity integration acknowledges that healthcare workers often define themselves through their ability to help others, creating conflicts when they need help themselves. Group work addresses these identity conflicts while maintaining positive aspects of professional identity that support healing.

Vicarious trauma processing recognizes that healthcare workers experience both direct trauma and secondary trauma through exposure to patient suffering. Treatment must address both types of trauma while building resilience for continued professional functioning.

Sarah, an emergency department nurse with a history of childhood sexual abuse, joined a healthcare worker trauma group after experiencing panic attacks during patient care situations that triggered her personal trauma memories. The group understood both her professional responsibilities and her personal healing needs.

The healthcare worker focus allowed discussion of professional triggers, strategies for managing trauma responses during work hours, and ways to maintain empathy for patients while protecting personal emotional boundaries.

Scheduling accommodations recognize that healthcare workers often have irregular schedules, mandatory overtime, and unpredictable work demands that affect therapy attendance. Flexible scheduling and make-up session options become essential for this population.

Religious and Spiritual Integration

Many trauma survivors find spiritual resources essential to their healing process, requiring thoughtful integration of religious and spiritual practices with evidence-based trauma treatment. These adaptations must respect diverse spiritual beliefs while avoiding inappropriate mixing of therapy and religious instruction.

Assessment of spiritual resources explores how individuals' faith traditions understand suffering, healing, and recovery while identifying spiritual practices that might support therapeutic goals. This assessment avoids making assumptions about spiritual beliefs while opening space for discussion of these often-important factors.

Collaboration with religious leaders when appropriate and desired by clients can provide additional support for trauma recovery while ensuring that therapy and spiritual guidance complement rather than conflict with each other.

Integration of spiritual practices might include prayer, meditation, scripture reading, or other practices that feel supportive to individual group members while maintaining respect for diverse beliefs within the group setting.

The case of Robert, an evangelical Christian dealing with combat trauma, illustrates spiritual integration challenges. His faith community viewed his PTSD symptoms as evidence of insufficient faith, creating additional shame and isolation that complicated his recovery process.

Spiritual reframing helped Robert understand his trauma symptoms as normal human responses to abnormal situations rather than spiritual failures. Discussions included how his faith could support rather than undermine his healing process while addressing the harmful messages he received from some community members.

Scripture integration included identifying biblical passages that supported healing and recovery while challenging interpretations that created additional shame or discouraged help-seeking. This work required collaboration with religious leaders who understood both trauma and theology.

The trauma group included members from different faith traditions, requiring careful facilitation to ensure that spiritual discussions remained supportive rather than divisive. Ground rules included respecting all sincere spiritual beliefs while focusing on how faith resources could support recovery rather than debating theological differences.

Secular adaptations ensure that individuals without religious beliefs or those from religious backgrounds who prefer secular treatment approaches can participate fully in group treatment without feeling excluded or pressured to adopt spiritual perspectives.

Language and Communication Adaptations

Language barriers create significant challenges for trauma group work while also providing opportunities for deeper cultural understanding and adaptation. These modifications address both practical communication needs and cultural meanings embedded in different languages.

Interpreter services require specialized training for interpreters working with trauma groups, including understanding of trauma symptoms, group dynamics, confidentiality requirements, and cultural factors that affect interpretation accuracy.

Bilingual group models may be more effective than interpreter-mediated groups for populations with sufficient numbers of individuals sharing the same language, allowing for more natural communication and cultural expression.

Language processing considerations recognize that trauma memories may be encoded in individuals' native languages, making processing in second languages less effective or emotionally meaningful.

The case of Carmen, a Spanish-speaking survivor of domestic violence, demonstrates language adaptation needs. Her trauma memories were encoded in Spanish, but her daily life occurred primarily in English, creating disconnection between her trauma experiences and her current coping resources.

Code-switching accommodation allowed Carmen to express trauma-related emotions in Spanish while learning coping strategies in English, honoring the language in which her experiences were encoded while building skills for her current environment.

Cultural concepts that don't translate directly required explanation and discussion to ensure accurate understanding. Terms like "personalismo," "simpatía," and "respeto" carried cultural meanings important to Carmen's healing but had no direct English equivalents.

The bilingual group model allowed for more natural expression of cultural values and healing concepts while providing peer support from others who shared both language and cultural background.

Written materials require translation that captures both literal meaning and cultural significance while maintaining therapeutic effectiveness. Simple translation often proves inadequate without cultural adaptation of concepts and examples.

Community and Family Involvement Strategies

Cultural groups vary significantly in their expectations about family involvement in individual problems, requiring flexible approaches that honor cultural values while maintaining therapeutic boundaries and individual autonomy.

Family assessment explores cultural expectations about family involvement while identifying family members who might support or interfere with individual healing. This assessment considers both nuclear and extended family relationships that may influence recovery.

Cultural mediation may be necessary when individual healing goals conflict with family expectations or cultural values, requiring skilled navigation that respects both individual autonomy and cultural belonging.

Community leader engagement can provide cultural guidance and community support for individuals participating in trauma treatment while addressing potential stigma or resistance within cultural communities.

The case of Fatima, a young Somali woman with sexual trauma history, illustrates family involvement challenges. Her participation in trauma treatment created conflict with family members who viewed her symptoms as bringing shame to the family and her treatment participation as evidence of weak faith.

Cultural education for family members helped them understand trauma symptoms as normal responses to abnormal experiences rather than character defects or spiritual failures. This education required

332

collaboration with trusted community leaders who could bridge cultural and clinical perspectives.

Gradual engagement started with education about trauma and healing within Islamic frameworks before introducing family members to therapeutic concepts and treatment approaches. This approach built understanding and support over time rather than creating immediate confrontation.

Gender considerations required sensitivity to cultural norms about mixed-gender interactions while ensuring that women had access to appropriate treatment. All-female groups with female facilitators felt more culturally appropriate for conservative religious communities.

Boundary negotiation helped Fatima maintain family relationships while protecting her individual healing process from family members who initially opposed her treatment participation.

The involvement of cultural brokers—trusted community members who understood both the culture and the treatment approach—proved invaluable for building family and community support for trauma treatment.

Community healing approaches recognize that individual trauma often occurs within contexts of community trauma, requiring interventions that address collective as well as individual healing needs.

Special Considerations for Marginalized Populations

Individuals from marginalized communities often experience trauma that intersects with oppression and discrimination, requiring adaptations that address both individual trauma and systemic factors that continue creating harm.

LGBTQ+ considerations include understanding how identity development, family rejection, and discrimination experiences create unique trauma presentations while recognizing diverse experiences within LGBTQ+ communities.

Microaggression awareness helps group facilitators recognize and address subtle forms of discrimination that might occur within group settings while building awareness among group members about how their words and actions affect others.

Intersectionality recognition acknowledges that individuals hold multiple identities that interact to create unique experiences of both oppression and resilience. African American transgender women, for example, face different challenges than white gay men, requiring individualized cultural understanding.

The case of Alex, a transgender man with childhood trauma history, illustrates LGBTQ+ considerations. His trauma included both childhood abuse and rejection by family members when he came out as transgender, creating complex grief and identity conflicts.

Affirming language included consistent use of chosen names and pronouns while creating group norms that supported all members' identities. Group agreements included education about respectful language and responses to mistakes or microaggressions.

Identity affirmation balanced processing of trauma experiences with celebration of identity strength and resilience. Treatment avoided pathologizing LGBTQ+ identities while addressing how discrimination and minority stress affected trauma recovery.

Community connection helped Alex build relationships with other LGBTQ+ individuals while finding chosen family relationships that provided support lacking from biological family members.

Safety planning included awareness of discrimination and violence risks while building strategies for managing identity disclosure decisions and maintaining physical and emotional safety.

The LGBTQ+ focus allowed for discussion of unique challenges while providing peer support from others who understood both trauma recovery and LGBTQ+ identity experiences.

Disability considerations ensure that trauma treatment remains accessible to individuals with physical, cognitive, or sensory disabilities while recognizing how disability experiences intersect with trauma histories.

Addressing Systemic Oppression

Individual trauma treatment must acknowledge systemic factors that contribute to trauma while providing support for both personal healing and community change efforts.

Power and privilege discussions help group members understand how social location affects trauma experiences while building awareness of both privilege and oppression that different members experience.

Historical trauma acknowledgment recognizes how collective trauma experiences affect individuals and communities across generations while providing frameworks for understanding individual symptoms within broader historical contexts.

Advocacy integration may include supporting group members' involvement in social justice activities while recognizing how advocacy work can both support and complicate individual healing processes.

Institutional analysis examines how systems like healthcare, education, criminal justice, and employment practices contribute to trauma while identifying strategies for navigating these systems more effectively.

The refugee trauma group addressed systemic factors including immigration policies, employment discrimination, and healthcare access barriers that affected group members' daily lives and trauma recovery.

Policy advocacy included supporting members' involvement in refugee rights organizations while providing emotional support for the stress and retraumatization that advocacy work sometimes creates.

Resource development involved connecting group members with legal services, job training programs, and community organizations that could address practical needs alongside mental health treatment.

Community organizing helped members find meaning and empowerment through working together to improve conditions for other refugees while building social connections and leadership skills.

Integration and Authenticity

The most effective cultural adaptations emerge from genuine collaboration between mental health professionals and cultural communities rather than superficial modifications that add cultural elements without understanding their deeper meanings.

Cultural humility requires ongoing learning, acknowledgment of limitations, and willingness to be corrected when cultural assumptions prove inaccurate. This humility builds trust while preventing harmful mistakes that can damage therapeutic relationships.

Authentic partnership involves cultural community members as consultants, supervisors, and collaborators in treatment development rather than simply as subjects of cultural adaptation efforts.

Continuous learning recognizes that cultural competence is an ongoing process rather than a fixed achievement, requiring regular education, consultation, and feedback from cultural community members.

The success of cultural adaptations depends on maintaining both cultural authenticity and therapeutic effectiveness while building bridges between different ways of understanding human suffering and healing.

Embracing Diversity in Healing

Cultural adaptations represent more than therapeutic techniques—they embody recognition that healing happens within cultural contexts and that effective treatment must honor the full complexity of human diversity. The goal is not to eliminate cultural differences but to create therapeutic spaces where diverse perspectives can coexist and contribute to collective healing.

These adaptations require ongoing commitment to learning, humility about limitations, and willingness to modify approaches based on feedback from cultural communities. The reward is treatment that feels authentic and effective for diverse populations while building cultural competence that benefits all participants.

Cultural Integration Essentials

- Cultural formulation examples demonstrate how cultural identity factors shape trauma presentation while informing culturally responsive treatment modifications
- Population-specific modifications honor unique cultural values while addressing specialized trauma presentations and healing expectations
- Religious and spiritual integration respects diverse faith traditions while incorporating spiritual resources that support therapeutic goals
- Language and communication adaptations address practical barriers while honoring cultural meanings embedded in different languages
- Community and family involvement strategies balance individual autonomy with cultural values about collective responsibility and support
- Addressing systemic oppression recognizes how social factors contribute to trauma while supporting both individual healing and community change efforts

Appendix E: Digital Resources and Technology Integration

Technology has become the invisible thread weaving through modern therapeutic practice—sometimes supporting and enhancing healing, other times creating barriers and complications that interfere with the human connections at the heart of recovery. This appendix provides practical guidance for integrating digital tools thoughtfully into trauma group work while avoiding the pitfalls that can turn helpful technology into technological hindrance.

The key lies in using technology to enhance rather than replace the fundamental human elements of healing while recognizing that different individuals have vastly different comfort levels, access, and interest in digital solutions.

QR Codes for Downloadable Materials

Quick Response (QR) codes provide immediate access to supplementary materials while bridging the gap between session content and daily life application. These digital doorways allow group members to access resources instantly without complicated website navigation or password management.

Implementation strategies involve placing QR codes on handouts and worksheets that link to audio versions of relaxation exercises, video demonstrations of grounding techniques, or downloadable forms for between-session practice. The codes should be large enough to scan easily while including backup website addresses for individuals who lack QR scanning capabilities.

Content libraries accessible through QR codes might include guided meditation recordings, trauma education videos, cultural resource materials, and crisis support information. These libraries should be regularly updated while maintaining stable links that won't frustrate users with broken connections.

Mobile optimization ensures that QR-linked content displays properly on smartphones and tablets while remaining accessible to individuals with varying levels of digital literacy. Simple, clean designs work better than complex interfaces that might overwhelm or confuse users.

The trauma group led by Dr. Martinez implemented QR codes that linked to audio recordings of group relaxation exercises, allowing members to practice techniques at home using the same voice and instructions from their group sessions. Usage data showed that 73% of group members accessed these resources at least weekly.

Privacy protection for QR-linked content requires secure hosting, encrypted connections, and clear privacy policies that protect user data while complying with healthcare privacy regulations. Users should understand what information is collected when they access digital resources.

Accessibility considerations include ensuring that QR-linked content works with screen readers and other assistive technologies used by individuals with disabilities. Alternative access methods should be available for those who cannot use QR codes.

Robert found QR codes particularly helpful because they eliminated the frustration of trying to remember website addresses or navigate complex online resources when he was feeling triggered or overwhelmed. The instant access allowed him to use coping strategies immediately when needed.

Usage tracking can provide valuable information about which resources are most helpful while identifying materials that might need updating or replacement. However, tracking should be implemented carefully to protect privacy and avoid creating surveillance anxiety.

Recommended Apps and Digital Tools

The mental health app marketplace includes thousands of options, but few have been rigorously tested with trauma populations. The recommendations here focus on evidence-based tools that complement group therapy while avoiding apps that might be triggering or harmful for trauma survivors.

Mood and symptom tracking apps like Daylio, eMoods, or Sanvello provide simple interfaces for monitoring daily emotional states, trigger exposure, and coping strategy effectiveness. These apps work best when integrated with group therapy through regular review of tracking data during sessions.

Selection criteria for mood tracking apps include user-friendly interfaces, data export capabilities, customizable categories that match therapeutic goals, and privacy protections that prevent unauthorized data sharing. Apps should enhance rather than burden the recovery process.

Mindfulness and meditation apps such as Headspace, Calm, or Insight Timer offer guided practices that can supplement group-learned techniques. However, trauma survivors may find some standard meditation practices triggering, requiring careful selection of trauma-informed mindfulness resources.

Crisis support apps like MY3, Safety Plan, or Crisis Text Line provide immediate access to safety resources while offering alternatives to emergency services for non-urgent situations. These apps should be introduced and practiced during stable periods rather than waiting for crisis situations.

The combat veteran group used the PTSD Coach app developed by the Department of Veterans Affairs, which includes trauma-specific coping strategies, symptom tracking, and direct connections to veteran crisis resources. Group members appreciated that the app was developed specifically for their population and experiences.

Grounding and coping apps like PTSD Coach, Breathe2Relax, or DBT Coach provide immediate access to regulation techniques while offering discrete support that can be used in public settings without drawing attention.

Jennifer found the Sanvello app helpful for tracking her anxiety levels and identifying patterns in her trigger responses. The data visualization helped her recognize that her symptoms followed predictable patterns related to her menstrual cycle and work stress, information that improved her self-understanding and coping planning.

Sleep support apps such as Sleep Cycle, Noisli, or Sleepio address the sleep disturbances that commonly accompany trauma while providing alternatives to medication-based approaches. Sleep tracking can reveal patterns that inform treatment planning.

Journaling apps like Day One, Journey, or Penzu offer secure platforms for written self-reflection while providing search capabilities and backup features that traditional paper journals lack. Some individuals find digital journaling more engaging than handwritten alternatives.

Telehealth Platform Comparisons

The rapid expansion of telehealth has created numerous platform options with varying features, security levels, and user experiences. Selecting appropriate platforms for trauma group work requires balancing functionality with privacy protection while considering diverse participant needs and preferences.

HIPAA-compliant platforms like Zoom for Healthcare, doxy.me, or SimplePractice Telehealth provide necessary privacy protections while offering features specifically designed for mental health services. Free platforms like standard Zoom or Skype typically lack adequate privacy protections for therapy use.

Group functionality varies significantly across platforms, with some offering robust group management features while others focus primarily on individual sessions. Important features include breakout rooms, screen sharing, recording capabilities, and participant management tools.

Accessibility features such as closed captioning, screen reader compatibility, and keyboard navigation become particularly important for trauma survivors who may have disabilities or who experience difficulty concentrating during triggered states.

User experience considerations include ease of joining sessions, technical support availability, and interface simplicity that doesn't create additional stress for individuals who may be struggling with concentration or technical challenges.

The refugee trauma group tested three different platforms before settling on Zoom for Healthcare, which provided the language interpretation features needed for their multilingual group while maintaining necessary privacy protections.

Security features should include end-to-end encryption, waiting rooms that prevent unauthorized access, and administrative controls that allow facilitators to manage participant behavior effectively.

Recording policies must balance the therapeutic benefits of session recordings with privacy concerns and legal requirements. Clear agreements about recording, storage, and access help prevent misunderstandings and privacy violations.

Maria appreciated that her telehealth platform allowed her to participate from home where she felt safer sharing vulnerable experiences, but she also found that technical difficulties sometimes interrupted emotional processing in ways that felt jarring and disruptive.

Technical support availability becomes crucial when technical problems occur during emotionally sensitive moments. Platforms should offer rapid support responses and backup communication methods when primary systems fail.

Technology Troubleshooting Guide

Technical problems inevitably occur during online therapy sessions, often at the worst possible moments when group members are sharing vulnerable content or processing difficult emotions. Proactive troubleshooting preparation can minimize disruptions while maintaining therapeutic momentum.

Common connectivity issues include poor internet connections, audio delays, video freezing, and complete disconnections that can disrupt group process and trigger anxiety in participants who may interpret technical problems as rejection or abandonment.

Preparation strategies involve testing all technology before sessions begin, having backup communication methods available, and establishing clear protocols for handling technical difficulties when they occur during sessions.

Audio problems frequently involve feedback, echo, or poor sound quality that makes communication difficult. Solutions include using headphones, muting when not speaking, and having phone backup options for individuals with persistent audio issues.

Video concerns might include poor lighting, distracting backgrounds, or camera positioning that affects communication quality. Virtual backgrounds can provide privacy while good lighting and camera positioning improve nonverbal communication.

The first responder trauma group developed a comprehensive troubleshooting protocol after multiple sessions were disrupted by technical difficulties that created additional stress for participants who were already struggling with hypervigilance and control issues.

Backup plans should include alternative communication methods like phone conferences, text messaging for brief communications, and clear procedures for rescheduling sessions when technical problems cannot be resolved quickly.

Participant support for technical difficulties includes providing written instructions for common problems, offering individual technical support sessions, and maintaining patience when repeated problems create frustration for technically challenged users.

David initially struggled with online group participation due to limited technical skills and older equipment. The program provided individual technical support and loaned him a tablet optimized for telehealth use, significantly improving his group experience.

Emergency protocols address what happens when technical failures occur during crisis situations, including alternative methods for ensuring safety and maintaining therapeutic relationships when primary communication methods fail.

Privacy and Security Considerations

Digital therapy tools create new privacy vulnerabilities that require careful attention to protect sensitive mental health information while maintaining the confidentiality that makes therapeutic relationships possible.

Data encryption ensures that information transmitted during online sessions cannot be intercepted or accessed by unauthorized individuals. End-to-end encryption provides the strongest protection while ensuring that even service providers cannot access session content.

Information storage policies should specify where and how session data is stored, who has access to stored information, how long information is retained, and how it is securely destroyed when no longer needed.

Third-party sharing agreements require careful review to understand what information may be shared with advertisers, researchers, or other organizations. Mental health apps often have complex privacy policies that users don't fully understand.

Device security involves protecting the phones, tablets, and computers used for therapy participation through password protection, automatic locking, and secure storage practices that prevent unauthorized access to sensitive information.

The women's trauma group discovered that one popular meditation app was sharing user data with advertising companies, leading to targeted ads for trauma-related products that felt intrusive and triggering for group members.

Home environment privacy requires ensuring that online therapy sessions cannot be overheard by family members, roommates, or others who might compromise confidentiality. This consideration becomes particularly important for individuals in unsafe or controlling relationships.

Professional boundaries may become blurred when therapy moves into participants' homes through technology. Clear agreements about session boundaries, appropriate dress, and environmental considerations help maintain therapeutic relationships.

Lisa had to relocate her online group participation to her car parked outside her house because her husband's work-from-home schedule made privacy impossible inside their small apartment. This solution worked but highlighted the complex logistics of maintaining confidentiality in online formats.

Cybersecurity threats including malware, phishing attempts, and hacking require basic digital security practices such as keeping software updated, using strong passwords, and avoiding suspicious links or downloads.

Digital Divide Considerations

Technology integration must address disparities in access, skills, and comfort levels that can exclude individuals from digital mental health resources while inadvertently creating additional barriers to treatment access.

Access disparities affect individuals who lack smartphones, computers, or reliable internet connections necessary for digital therapy participation. These disparities often correlate with economic disadvantage that already creates barriers to mental health treatment.

Digital literacy varies widely among potential group members, with some individuals feeling comfortable with advanced technology while others struggle with basic smartphone functions. Training and support must be available to bridge these skill gaps.

Economic barriers include not only device and internet costs but also data plan limitations that might restrict video calling or downloading of therapy resources. Unlimited data plans often cost more than economically disadvantaged individuals can afford.

Age-related differences in technology comfort and skills require flexible approaches that don't exclude older adults who might benefit from group treatment but feel intimidated by digital participation requirements.

The refugee trauma group addressed digital divide issues by partnering with a local library system that provided free internet access and basic technology training while lending tablets to participants who lacked appropriate devices.

Cultural factors may influence technology acceptance and use patterns, with some cultural groups viewing digital therapy as less legitimate or trustworthy than in-person services. Cultural education and adaptation can help address these concerns.

Disability accommodations ensure that digital resources work with assistive technologies used by individuals with visual, hearing, or motor impairments while providing alternative access methods when standard digital tools are inaccessible.

Rural connectivity challenges include limited internet infrastructure, data plan restrictions, and technology service limitations that affect individuals in remote areas who may have limited access to in-person mental health services.

Michael lived in a rural area with spotty internet service that made video group participation unreliable. The program developed a hybrid approach where he participated by phone during internet outages while maintaining video connection when possible, ensuring consistent access regardless of connectivity issues.

Family technology sharing situations require consideration of privacy when multiple family members share devices or internet connections. Solutions might include headphones for privacy, scheduling around family technology use, or providing individual devices when possible.

Integration Best Practices

Successful technology integration requires thoughtful planning, ongoing evaluation, and flexibility to adapt digital tools based on user feedback and changing needs. The goal is enhancing rather than complicating the therapeutic process.

Gradual implementation introduces digital tools slowly while building comfort and skills over time rather than overwhelming participants with multiple new technologies simultaneously. Start with simple, user-friendly tools before advancing to more complex applications.

User choice allows individuals to select which digital tools feel helpful while avoiding pressure to use technology that creates stress or feels intrusive. Not everyone benefits from the same digital approaches, requiring individualized selection and implementation.

Training and support should be readily available for all digital tools used in therapy while recognizing that ongoing support may be needed as individuals' comfort levels and technology skills develop over time.

Regular evaluation assesses whether digital tools are achieving their intended purposes while identifying tools that create more problems than benefits. Technology should be modified or discontinued when it interferes with therapeutic goals.

The healthcare worker trauma group evaluated their technology use quarterly, discontinuing apps that participants found burdensome while expanding use of tools that provided genuine benefit. This ongoing evaluation ensured that technology served rather than dominated the therapeutic process.

Backup options ensure that therapy can continue when technology fails while maintaining therapeutic relationships and progress even when digital tools become unavailable. Low-tech alternatives should always be available.

Privacy education helps participants understand digital privacy risks while teaching practical skills for protecting sensitive information. This education empowers informed decision-making about technology use rather than creating technology avoidance.

Jennifer learned to adjust her social media privacy settings after realizing that her participation in trauma treatment might be visible to family members who didn't know about her therapy involvement. The education helped her maintain both treatment engagement and family privacy.

Cost-benefit analysis regularly evaluates whether the benefits of digital tools justify their costs in terms of money, time, and emotional energy while ensuring that technology enhances rather than burdens the recovery process.

Future Technology Trends

Emerging technologies offer new possibilities for trauma treatment while raising additional questions about privacy, effectiveness, and appropriate integration with human therapeutic relationships.

Artificial intelligence applications might include personalized coping strategy recommendations, risk assessment support, or automated screening tools that enhance but don't replace human clinical judgment.

Virtual reality therapeutic applications continue expanding beyond exposure therapy to include safe environment creation, social skills practice, and immersive relaxation experiences that might enhance group therapy approaches.

Wearable devices provide objective data about stress levels, sleep patterns, and physical activity that could inform treatment planning while offering biofeedback for nervous system regulation training.

Predictive analytics might eventually identify individuals at risk for crisis or dropout while suggesting interventions that prevent problems before they become severe.

The trauma research consortium is exploring virtual reality applications that allow group members to practice difficult conversations or challenging situations in safe virtual environments before attempting them in real life.

Biometric integration through smartwatches or fitness trackers could provide real-time data about heart rate variability, sleep quality, and activity levels that inform understanding of treatment progress and daily functioning patterns.

Voice analysis technology might eventually detect emotional states or crisis risk through speech pattern analysis, though privacy and accuracy concerns require careful consideration before clinical implementation.

Robert participated in a pilot study using smartwatch data to track his sleep patterns and physical activity, revealing correlations between his exercise routine and trauma symptom severity that informed his treatment planning and self-care strategies.

Blockchain technology offers potential solutions for secure health data sharing while maintaining privacy and giving individuals control over their personal information access and use.

Ethical Technology Use

Technology integration in trauma treatment raises important ethical questions about privacy, effectiveness, informed consent, and the appropriate balance between digital tools and human therapeutic relationships.

Informed consent for technology use must address data collection, storage, sharing practices, and potential risks while ensuring that participants understand what they're agreeing to when using digital mental health tools.

Professional competence requires therapists to understand the technology they recommend while staying informed about privacy practices, effectiveness research, and potential risks associated with digital tools.

Boundary considerations become complex when technology creates new forms of contact between therapists and clients or when digital tools blur the boundaries between therapy sessions and daily life.

Quality assurance involves evaluating digital tools for safety, effectiveness, and appropriate use while avoiding recommendation of products that haven't been adequately tested or that might be harmful for trauma populations.

The ethics committee at Maria's treatment center developed guidelines for technology recommendation that required evidence of effectiveness, privacy protection, and appropriate informed consent before therapists could recommend specific apps or digital tools to clients.

Cultural sensitivity in technology use considers how different populations relate to digital tools while ensuring that technology integration doesn't create additional barriers for culturally diverse participants.

Digital equity efforts work to ensure that technology enhances rather than limits access to mental health services while addressing disparities that might exclude economically disadvantaged individuals from digital health resources.

Bridging Digital and Human Healing

Technology at its best serves as a bridge that extends the healing power of human connection beyond the boundaries of scheduled sessions and therapy offices. The most effective digital tools enhance rather than replace the fundamental human elements of empathy, understanding, and authentic relationship that make healing possible.

The challenge lies in using technology thoughtfully and purposefully while maintaining the human-centered focus that defines effective trauma treatment. Digital tools should feel like natural extensions of therapeutic relationships rather than cold, impersonal substitutes for human connection.

The future of trauma treatment will likely include increasing technology integration, but the heart of healing will remain fundamentally human—requiring presence, understanding, and the courage to witness and support each other through the difficult journey from survival to thriving.

Technology Implementation Framework

- QR codes provide immediate access to supplementary materials while bridging session content with daily life application through mobile-optimized resources
- Recommended apps and digital tools should be evidence-based and trauma-informed while addressing specific therapeutic goals and user privacy needs
- Telehealth platform selection requires balancing functionality with privacy protection while considering diverse participant needs and accessibility requirements

- Technology troubleshooting guides minimize session disruptions while maintaining therapeutic momentum during technical difficulties
- Privacy and security considerations protect sensitive mental health information while maintaining the confidentiality essential for therapeutic relationships
- Digital divide awareness ensures equitable access while addressing disparities in technology access, skills, and comfort levels across diverse populations

Reference

1. van der Kolk, B. A. (2014). *The body keeps the score: Brain, mind, and body in the healing of trauma.* Viking.
2. Siegel, D. J. (1999). *The developing mind: How relationships and the brain interact to shape who we are.* Guilford Press.
3. Felitti, V. J., Anda, R. F., Nordenberg, D., Williamson, D. F., Spitz, A. M., Edwards, V., & Marks, J. S. (1998). Relationship of childhood abuse and household dysfunction to many of the leading causes of death in adults: The Adverse Childhood Experiences (ACE) Study. *American Journal of Preventive Medicine*, 14(4), 245-258.
4. Weathers, F. W., Blake, D. D., Schnurr, P. P., Kaloupek, D. G., Marx, B. P., & Keane, T. M. (2013). *The Clinician-Administered PTSD Scale for DSM-5 (CAPS-5).* National Center for PTSD.
5. Briere, J. (2011). *Trauma Symptom Inventory-2 (TSI-2): Professional manual.* Psychological Assessment Resources.
6. Cloitre, M., Shevlin, M., Brewin, C. R., Bisson, J. I., Roberts, N. P., Maercker, A., ... & Hyland, P. (2018). The International Trauma Questionnaire: Development of a self-report measure of ICD-11 PTSD and complex PTSD. *Journal of Traumatic Stress*, 31(6), 803-817.
7. Bernstein, E. M., & Putnam, F. W. (1986). Development, reliability, and validity of a dissociation scale. *Journal of Nervous and Mental Disease*, 174(12), 727-735.
8. Young, J. E., Klosko, J. S., & Weishaar, M. E. (2003). *Schema therapy: A practitioner's guide.* Guilford Press.
9. Porges, S. W. (2011). *The polyvagal theory: Neurophysiological foundations of emotions, attachment, communication, and self-regulation.* Norton.
10. Dana, D. (2018). *The polyvagal theory in therapy: Engaging the rhythm of regulation.* Norton.
11. Sloan, D. M., Feinstein, B. A., Gallagher, M. W., Beck, J. G., & Keane, T. M. (2013). Efficacy of group treatment for posttraumatic stress disorder symptoms: A meta-analysis. *Psychological Trauma: Theory, Research, Practice, and Policy*, 5(2), 176-183.

12. Yalom, I. D., & Leszcz, M. (2020). *The theory and practice of group psychotherapy* (6th ed.). Basic Books.

13. Kitchiner, N. J., Lewis, C., Roberts, N. P., & Bisson, J. I. (2019). Active duty and ex-serving military personnel with PTSD treated with psychological therapies: A systematic review and meta-analysis. *European Journal of Psychotraumatology*, 10(1), 1684226.

14. Farrell, J. M., Shaw, I. A., & Webber, M. A. (2009). A schema-focused approach to group psychotherapy for outpatients with borderline personality disorder: A randomized controlled trial. *Journal of Behavior Therapy and Experimental Psychiatry*, 40(2), 317-328.

15. Young, J. E. (2005). *Young Schema Questionnaire–Short Form 3 (YSQ-S3)*. Schema Therapy Institute.

16. McCraty, R., Atkinson, M., Tomasino, D., & Bradley, R. T. (2009). The coherent heart: Heart-brain interactions, psychophysiological coherence, and the emergence of system-wide order. *Integral Review*, 5(2), 10-115.

17. Levine, P. A. (2010). *In an unspoken voice: How the body releases trauma and restores goodness*. North Atlantic Books.

18. Schwartz, R. C. (2021). *No bad parts: Healing trauma and restoring wholeness with the Internal Family Systems model*. Sounds True.

19. Gilbert, P. (2009). *The compassionate mind: A new approach to life's challenges*. Constable & Robinson.

20. McCann, I. L., & Pearlman, L. A. (1990). Vicarious traumatization: A framework for understanding the psychological effects of working with victims. *Journal of Traumatic Stress*, 3(1), 131-149.

21. Figley, C. R. (2002). Compassion fatigue: Psychotherapists' chronic lack of self care. *Journal of Clinical Psychology*, 58(11), 1433-1441.

22. Stamm, B. H. (2010). *The concise ProQOL manual* (2nd ed.). ProQOL.org.

23. Newell, J. M., & MacNeil, G. A. (2010). Professional burnout, vicarious trauma, secondary traumatic stress, and compassion fatigue: A review of the literature. *Clinical Social Work Journal*, 38(3), 319-338.

24. Substance Abuse and Mental Health Services Administration. (2014). *Trauma-informed care in behavioral services.* Treatment Improvement Protocol (TIP) Series 57. HHS Publication No. (SMA) 13-4801.
25. National Child Traumatic Stress Network. (2011). *Secondary traumatic stress: A fact sheet for child-serving professionals.* Los Angeles, CA & Durham, NC: Author.
26. Kadambi, M. A., & Truscott, D. (2004). Vicarious trauma among therapists working with sexual violence, cancer, and general practice. *Canadian Journal of Counselling*, 38(4), 260-276.
27. Adams, R. E., Boscarino, J. A., & Figley, C. R. (2006). Compassion fatigue and psychological distress among social workers: A validation study. *American Journal of Orthopsychiatry*, 76(1), 103-108.
28. Tedeschi, R. G., & Calhoun, L. G. (2004). Posttraumatic growth: Conceptual foundations and empirical evidence. *Psychological Inquiry*, 15(1), 1-18.
29. Joseph, S., & Linley, P. A. (2005). Positive adjustment to threatening events: An organismic valuing theory of growth through adversity. *Review of General Psychology*, 9(3), 262-280.
30. Farrell, J. M., Shaw, I. A., & Webber, M. A. (2009). A schema-focused approach to group psychotherapy for outpatients with borderline personality disorder: A randomized controlled trial. *Journal of Behavior Therapy and Experimental Psychiatry*, 40(2), 317-328.
31. Sempertegui, G. A., Karreman, A., Arntz, A., & Bekker, M. H. (2013). Schema therapy for borderline personality disorder: A comprehensive review of its empirical foundations, effectiveness and implementation possibilities. *Clinical Psychology Review*, 33(3), 426-447.
32. Sloan, D. M., Feinstein, B. A., Gallagher, M. W., Beck, J. G., & Keane, T. M. (2013). Efficacy of group treatment for posttraumatic stress disorder symptoms: A meta-analysis. *Psychological Trauma: Theory, Research, Practice, and Policy*, 5(2), 176-183.

33. Ehlers, A., & Clark, D. M. (2000). A cognitive model of posttraumatic stress disorder. *Behaviour Research and Therapy*, 38(4), 319-345.
34. Van Asselt, A. D., Dirksen, C. D., Arntz, A., & Severens, J. L. (2007). The cost of borderline personality disorder: Societal cost of illness in BPD-patients. *European Psychiatry*, 22(6), 354-361.
35. Nordahl, H. M., & Nysaeter, T. E. (2005). Schema therapy for patients with borderline personality disorder: A single case series. *Journal of Behavior Therapy and Experimental Psychiatry*, 36(4), 254-264.
36. Bamelis, L. L., Evers, S. M., Spinhoven, P., & Arntz, A. (2014). Results of a multicenter randomized controlled trial of the clinical effectiveness of schema therapy for personality disorders. *American Journal of Psychiatry*, 171(3), 305-322.
37. Bamelis, L. L., Evers, S. M., Spinhoven, P., & Arntz, A. (2014). Results of a multicenter randomized controlled trial of the clinical effectiveness of schema therapy for personality disorders. *American Journal of Psychiatry*, 171(3), 305-322.

www.ingramcontent.com/pod-product-compliance
Lightning Source LLC
Chambersburg PA
CBHW071640280326
41928CB00068B/1802